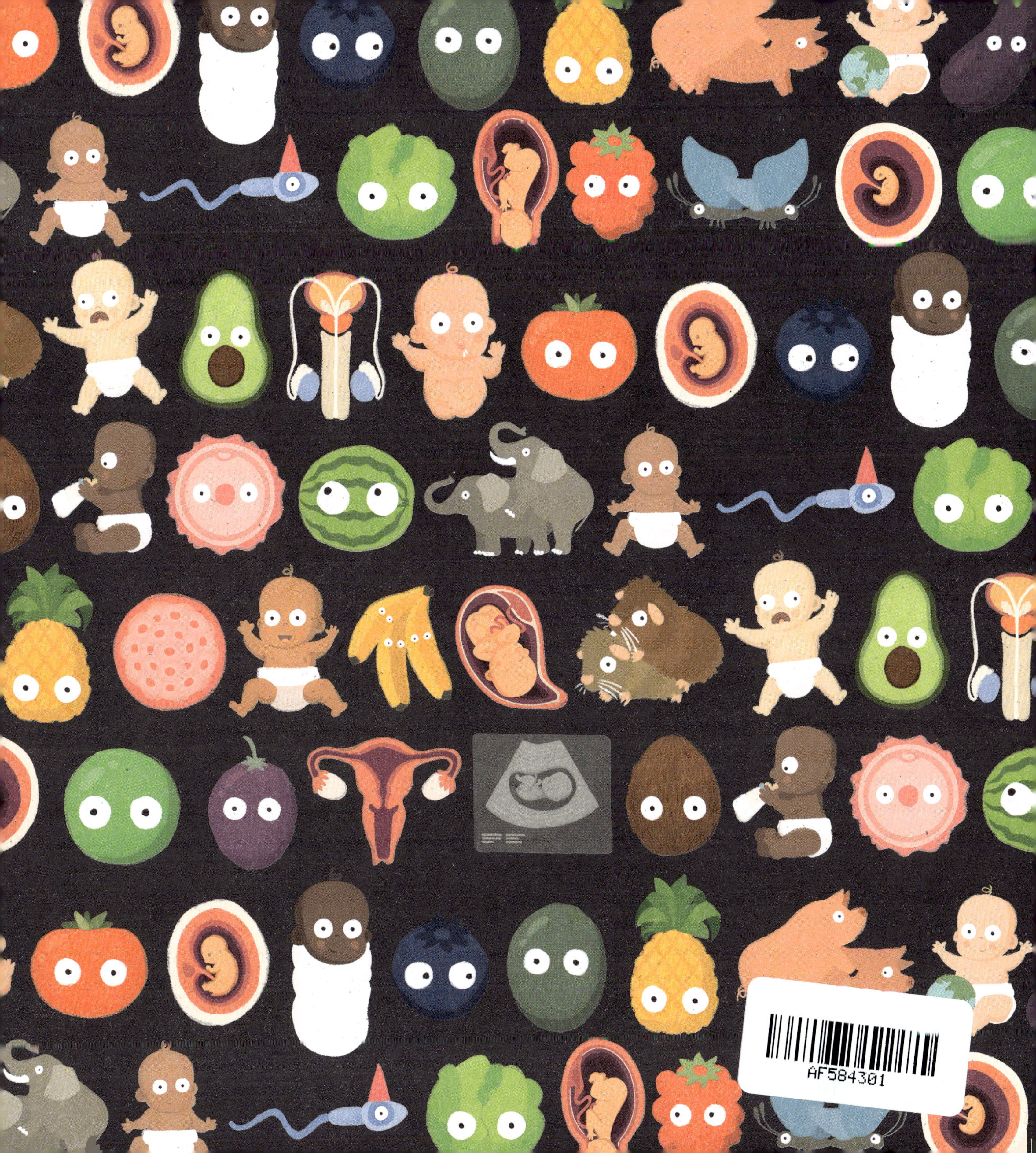

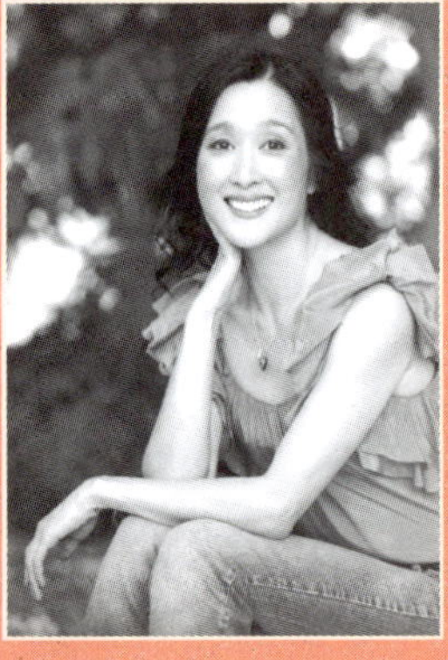

Foreword.

Dear Parent or Caregiver,

Congratulations! You are taking a valuable step in demystifying one of the most potentially confusing human functions: conception and pregnancy.

Being willing to call a spade a spade (and a uterus a uterus) can be vitally important when it comes to helping kids understand how their bodies function, and especially in promoting a sound conception of conception. Euphemisms can lead to confusion and misunderstanding, as I discovered, with blinding clarity, many moons ago.

One merry afternoon, my three-year-old quite unexpectedly piped up, 'How does sperm get into a woman's tummy? How does she eat it?' he mused, whilst miming trying to eat an object the size of a softball.

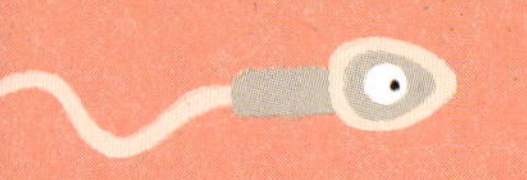

'Hang on, what do you mean?' I asked.

'Well,' Master Three explained in an exasperated tone, 'to grow the baby in your tummy, you obviously have to eat the sperm! That's how it gets into your tummy, right?'

'I can see where you're coming from, but the baby doesn't actually grow in the tummy. The "tummy" is your stomach, where the food goes, but the baby actually grows in a different place.'

'What? You have a separate tummy in your tummy?'

'Not really. Lower down, here, in this area called the pelvis, women have a special bag called the uterus, and that's where the baby actually grows.'

Master Three looked mildly sceptical. 'So, how does it get in there?'

'Well, there's actually an opening down here with a passage that leads up to the uterus. It's called the vagina.'

'For-China,' he mused, then with a flash of inspiration added, 'Yes, that's why we're Chinese . . . your Mum is from China, you're from her "for China" and I'm from your "for China!"'

'Umm, no, it's va-gina. Not *China.* But yeah, I see where you're coming from . . .'

This book demonstrates how babies are made in a manner that is delightful to behold, as well as extremely easy to understand. Kids will find the book fun to read, either autonomously or with a trusted adult. It is effortlessly educational, engaging and entertaining.

Pictures paint a thousand words and will help young people not confuse vagina with 'for China' and vulvas with Volvos (a story for another time!), and, perhaps most importantly, will distinguish the uterus from that vague all-purpose catch-all, the 'tummy'.

May all the parents, carers, teachers and grandparents enjoy using this wonderful resource to help untangle the confusion around one of life's most fascinating and mysterious of miracles.

Cindy

Dr Cindy Pan MBBS, FRACGP
cindypan.com.au

How babies are made.

PHILIP BUNTING

Just like most other animals, we hairy humans make babies through a nifty little process known as Sexual Reproduction.

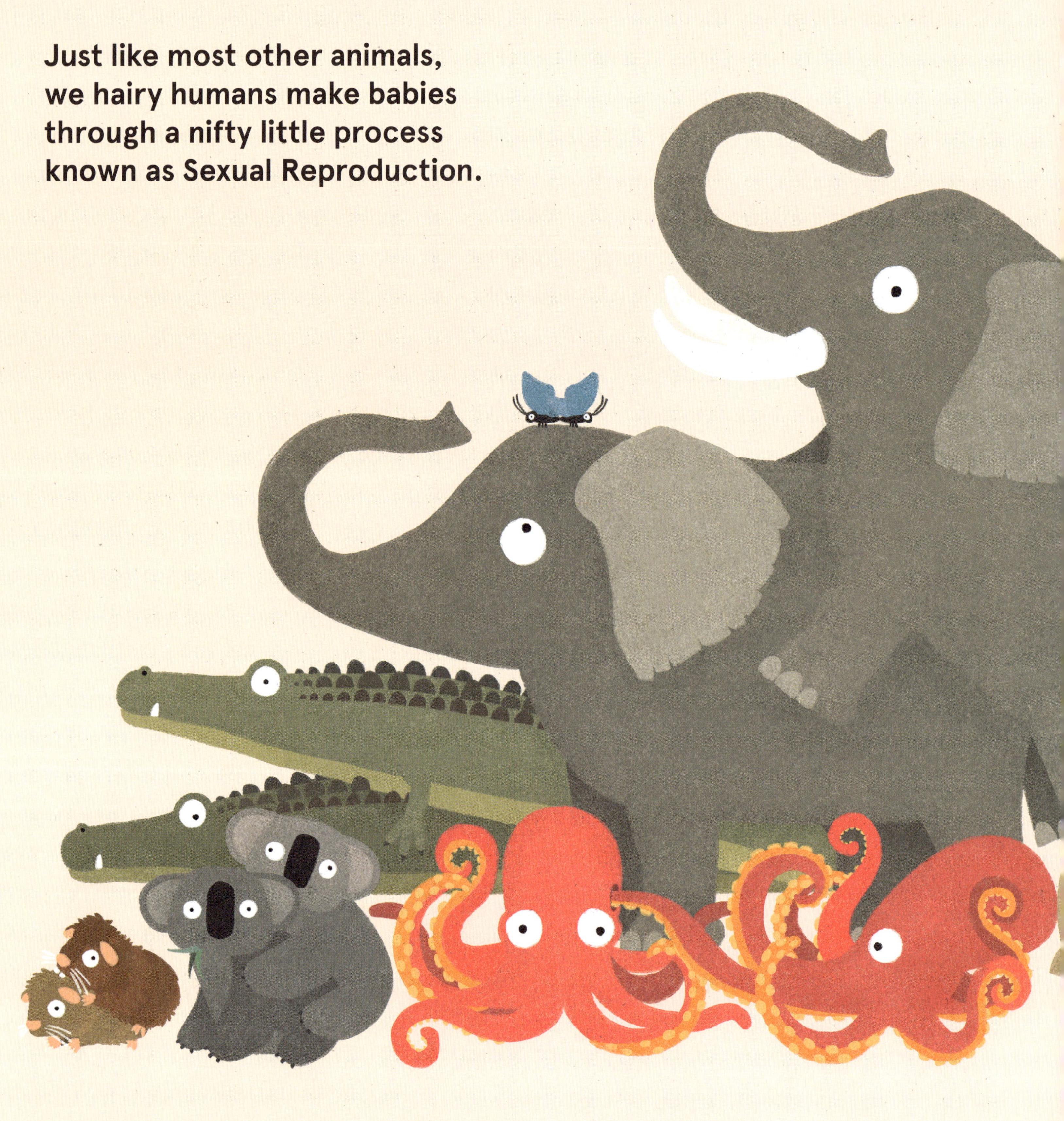

This requires two participants: a biological male and a biological female from the same species (*Homo sapiens*, in our case).

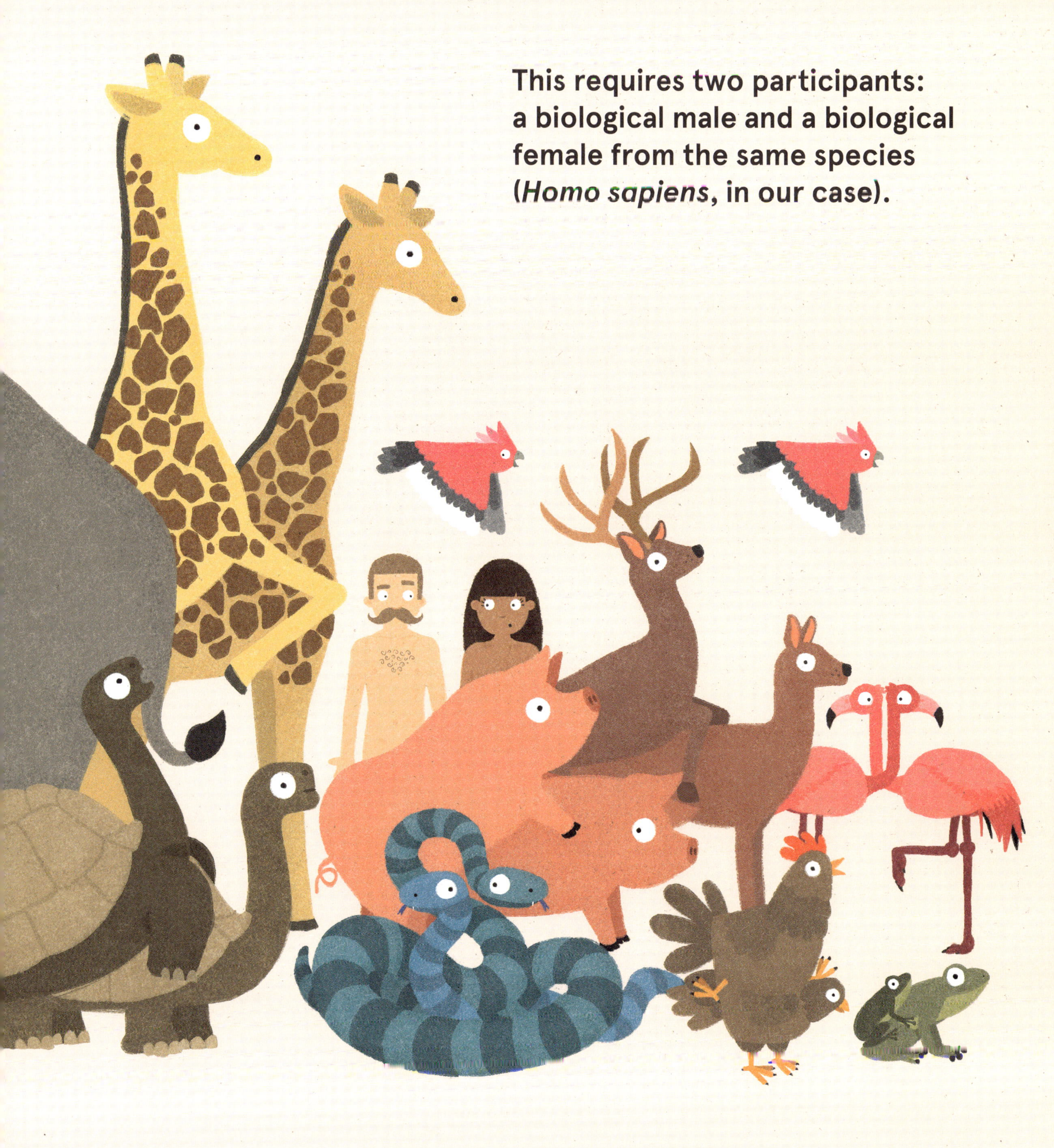

We humans are all pretty similar to one another. The things that make us alike vastly outnumber the things that make us different.

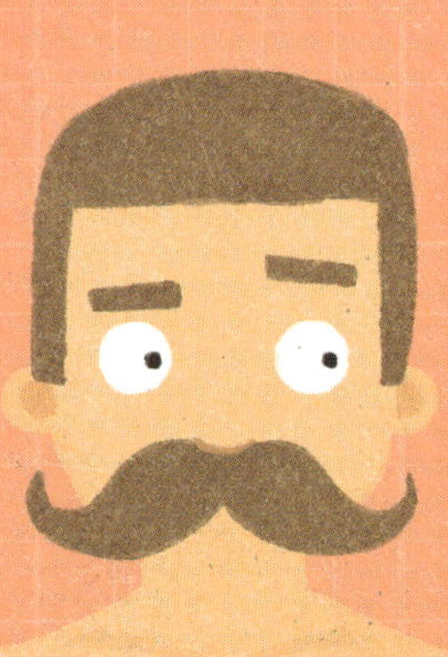

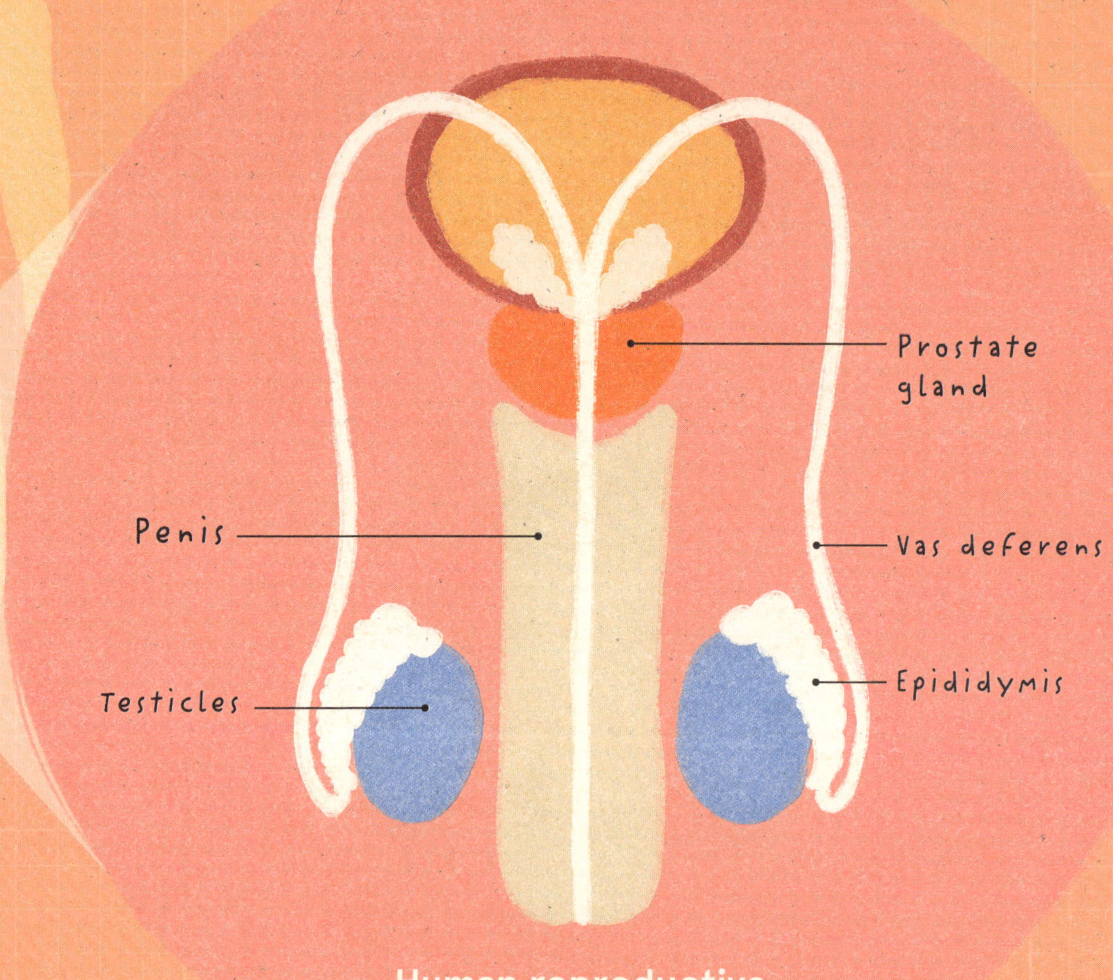

Human reproductive system (male).

Perhaps the most noticeable differences between most male and female humans can be found in the bits that help us to make babies.

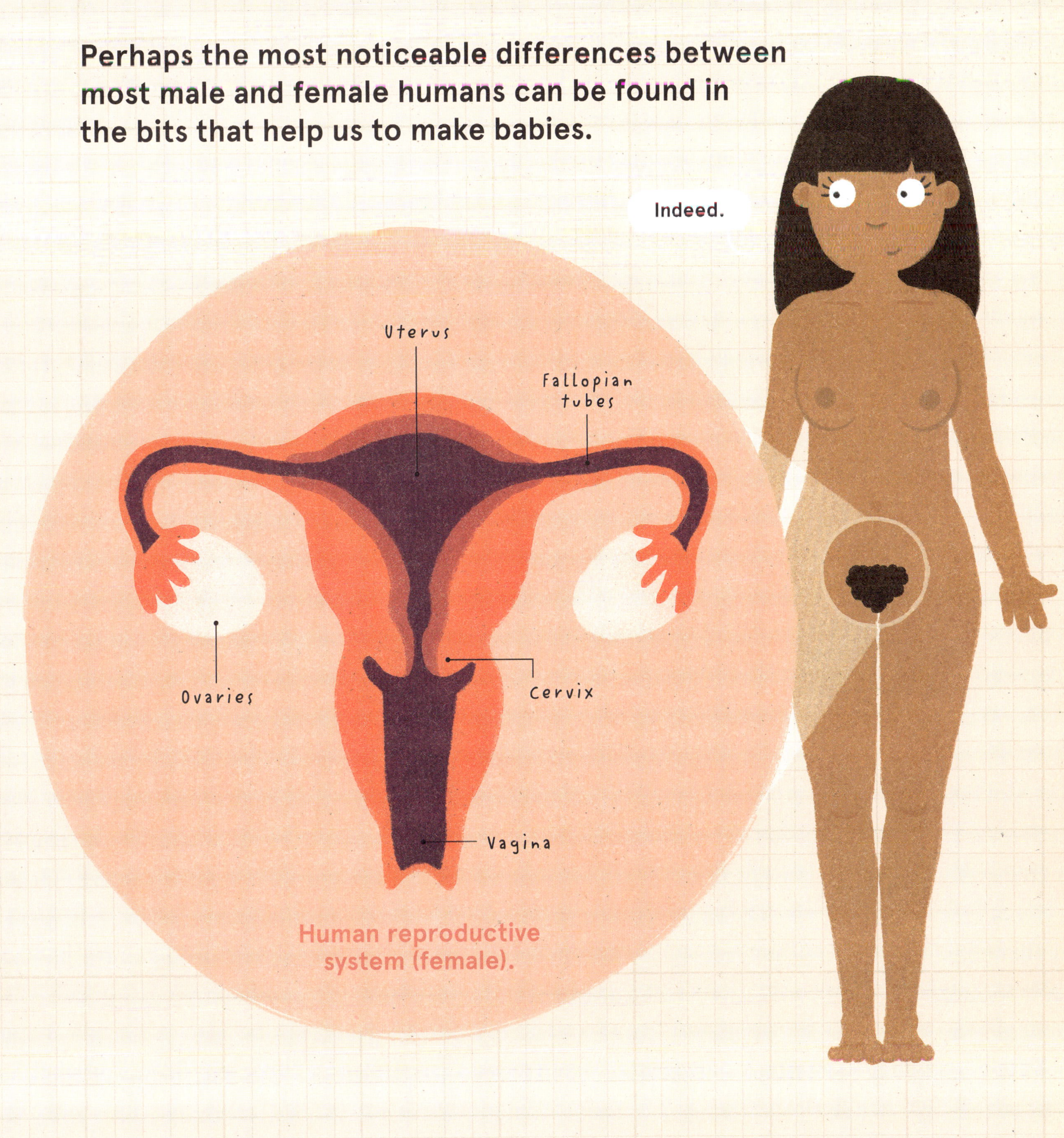

Human reproductive system (female).

Once we reach adulthood, most male humans create a special kind of cell in their testicles, called sperm.

Spermatozoa.

(or 'sperm')

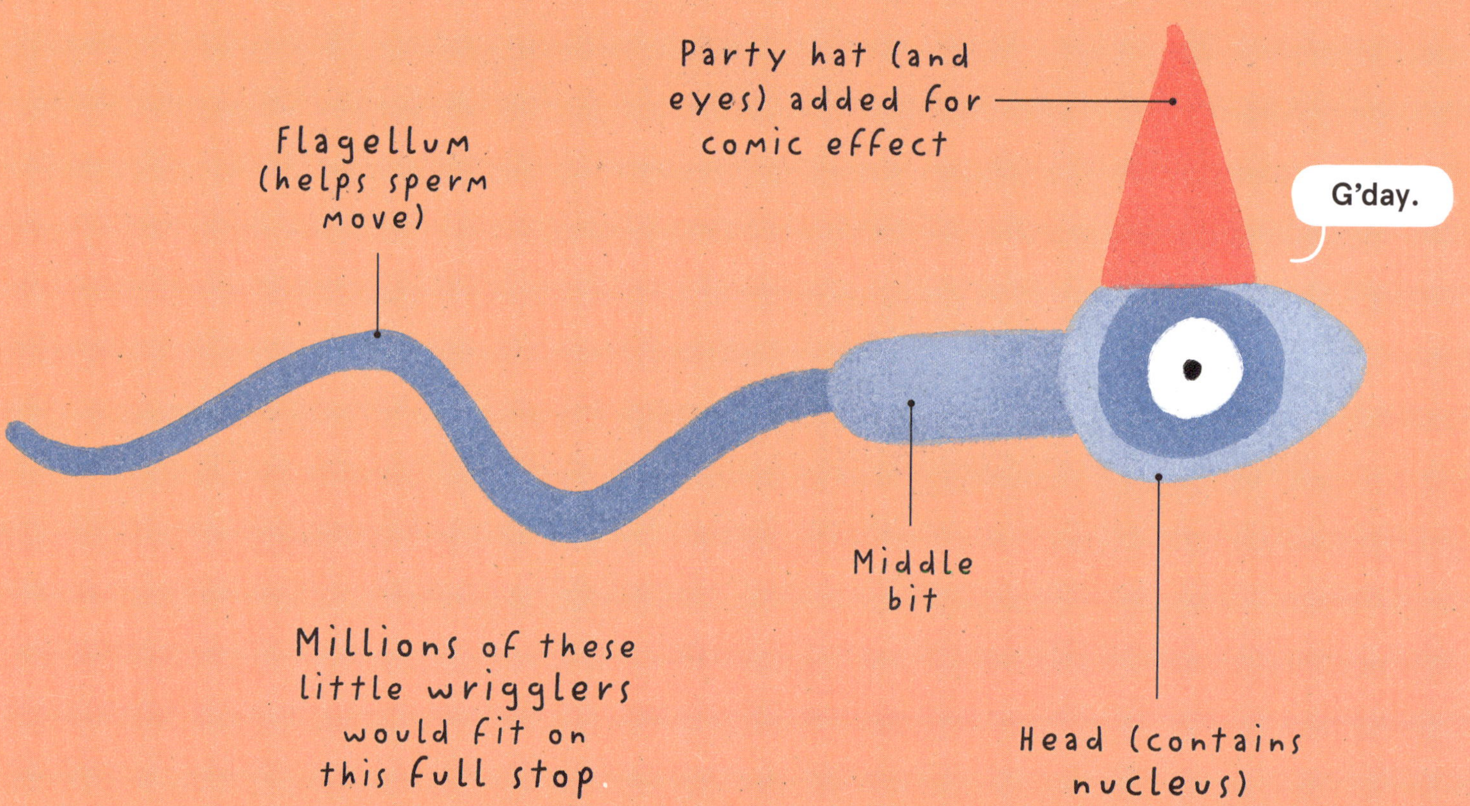

Millions of these little wrigglers would fit on this full stop.

Sperm are a bit like a tiny living seed, with a head and a tadpole-like tail (but no eyes, and certainly no party hat).

Females typically create a special kind of cell in their ovaries, called ovum. An ovum is a bit like a soft little egg.

Ovum.

(or 'egg')

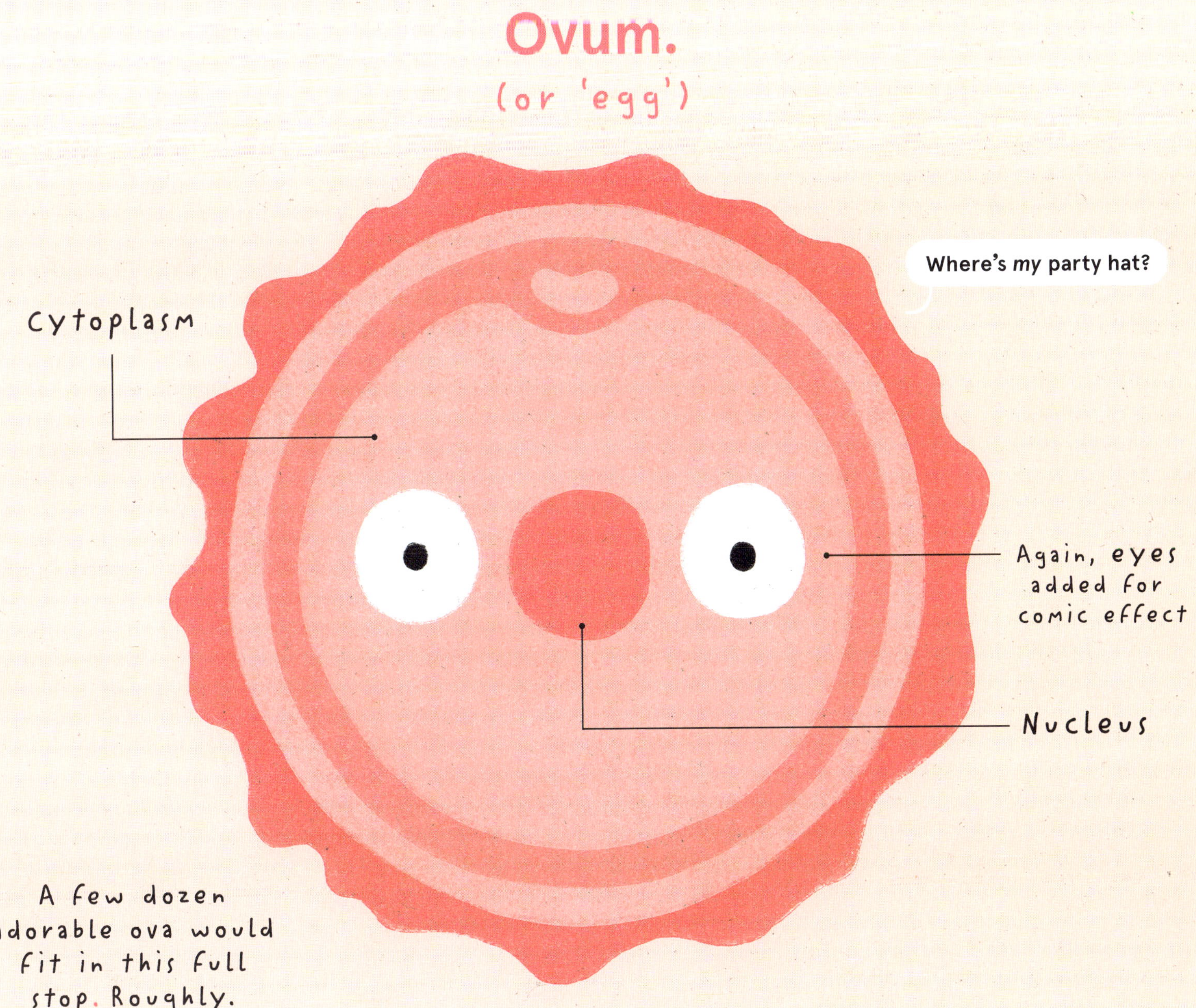

A few dozen adorable ova would fit in this full stop. Roughly.

An ovum is about 10 million times the volume of a sperm cell (yet they're still very, very tiny).

To make a brand-new human, you need one sperm cell and one egg cell.

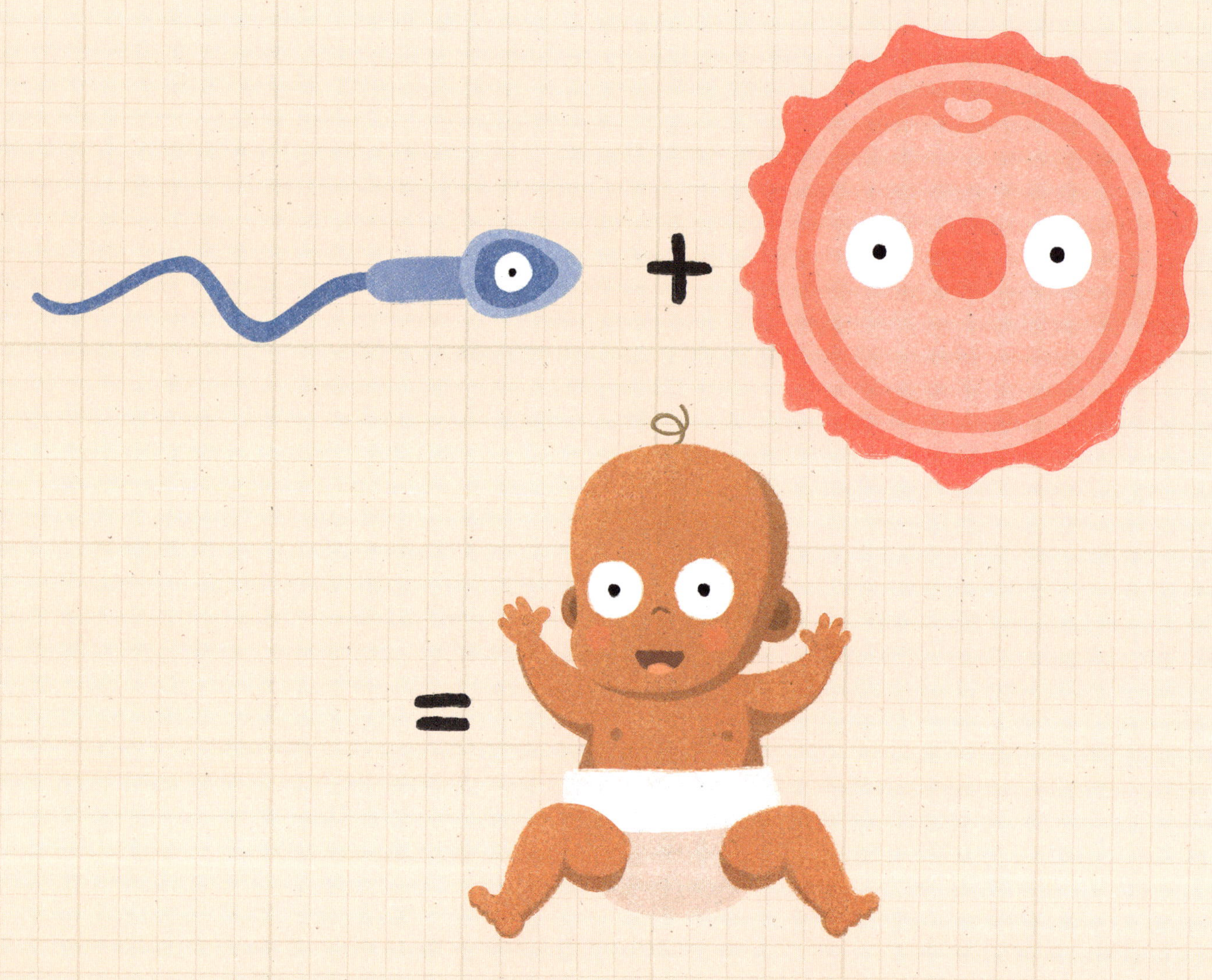

The sperm and egg must meet, then join together to become the beginnings of a baby. So how do they meet?

Strap in.

Sometimes – when the mood is *just right*, and the stars align, and a twinkle flashes between their eyes – two adults will take part in an activity we know as Sexual Intercourse.

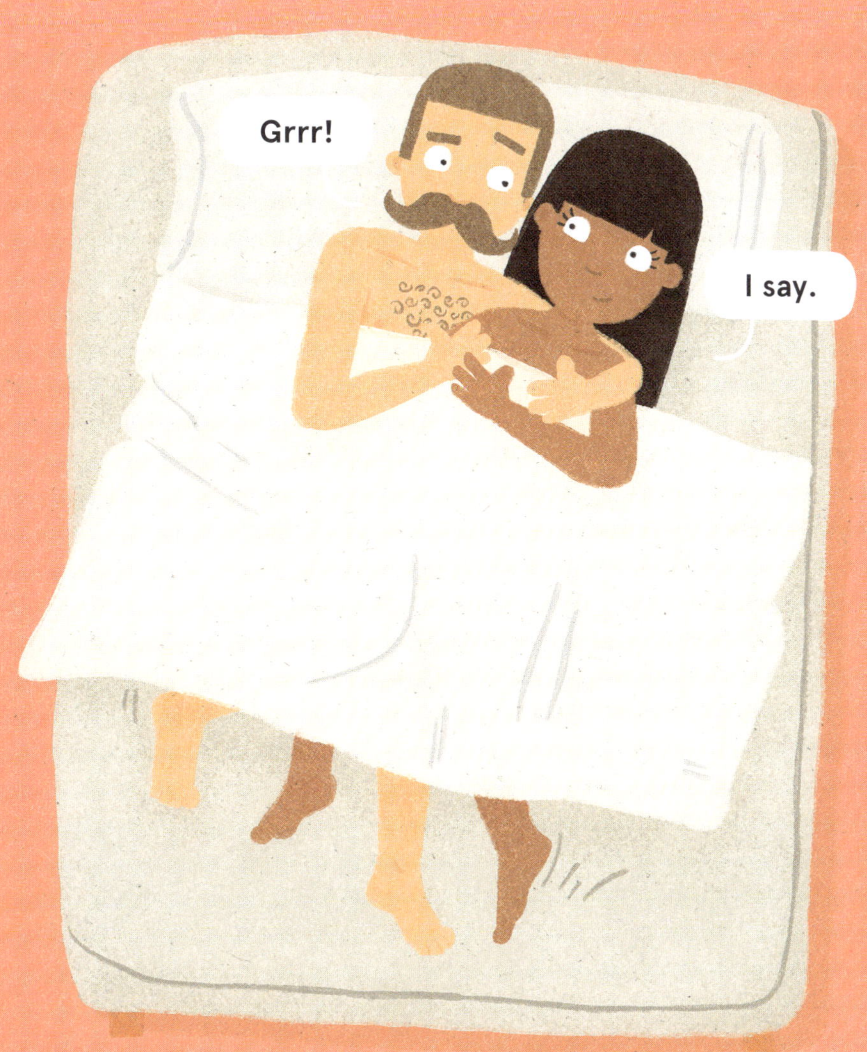

During this jolly jaunt, the male's brain sends signals to his penis, which becomes stiff and points forward.

When the adult female lets him know to do so, the adult male puts his penis inside the female's vagina. Like so ...

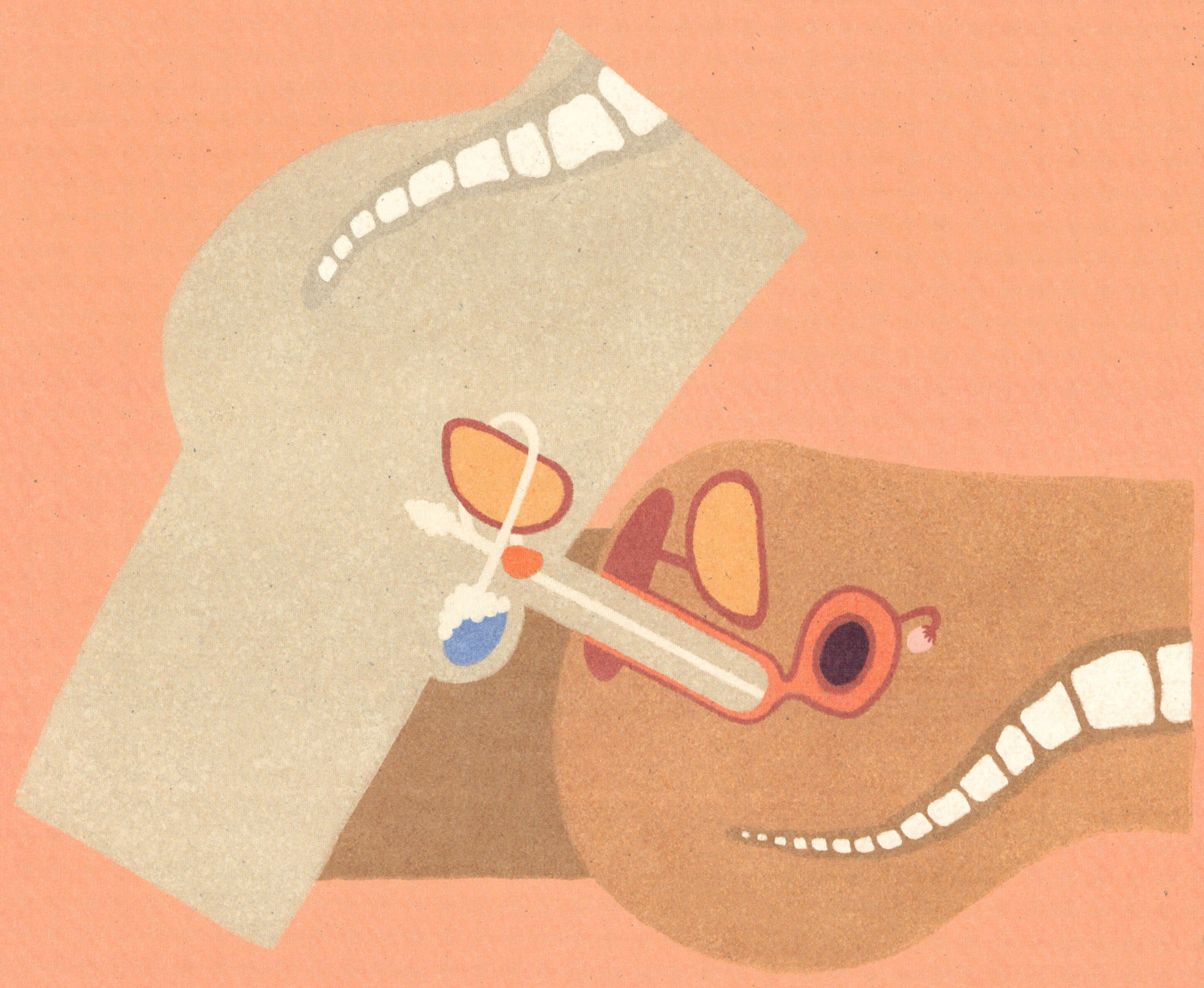

After some wiggling, wriggling and perhaps a little bit of jiggling, the male's body gives his reproductive organs a signal ...

and in pretty short order, millions of sperm cells are released from his epididymis. From there, they travel along the penis, out of the male's body and into the female's.

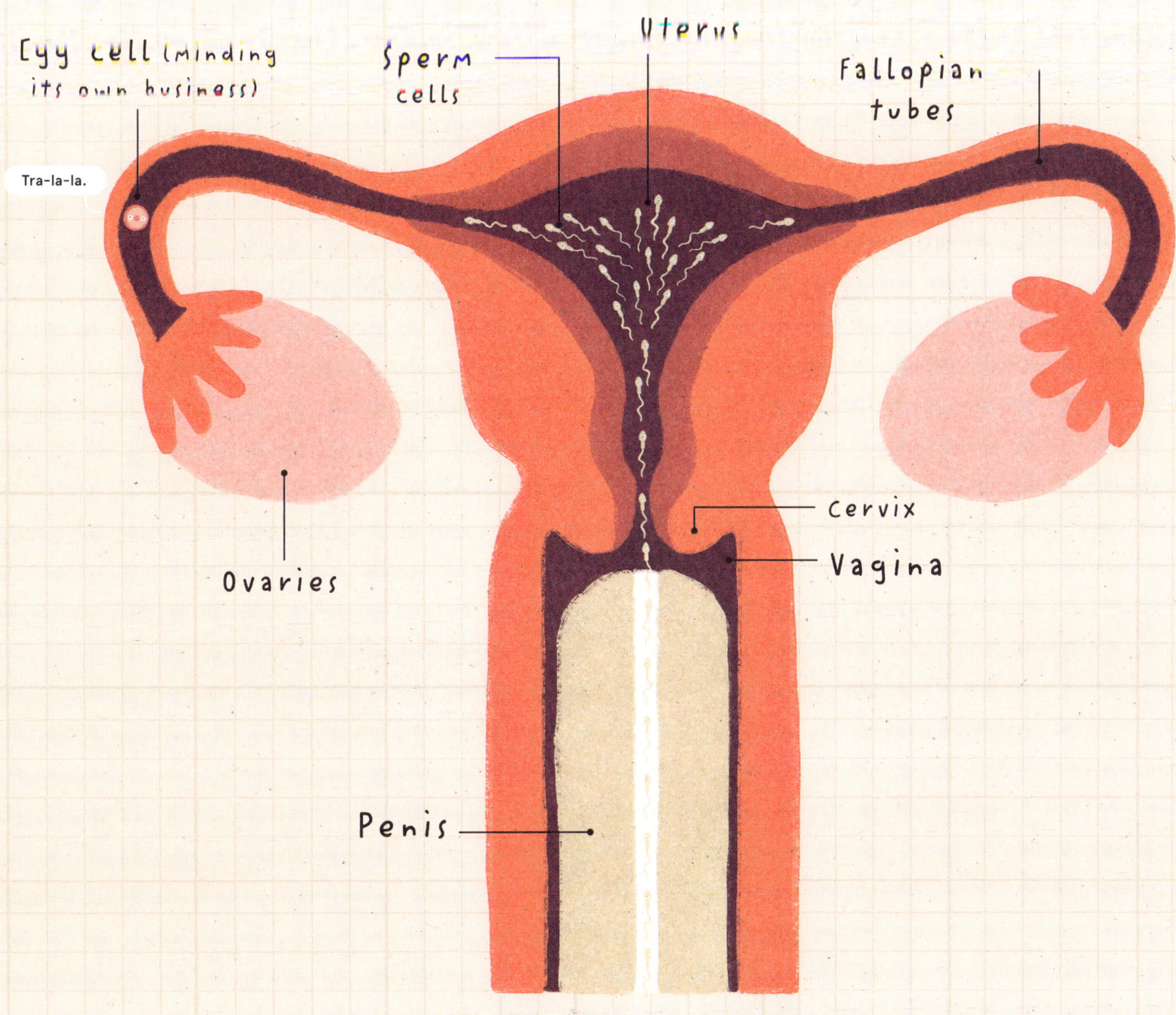

The sperm cells use their tails to swim up through the vagina, past the cervix, through the uterus and into the fallopian tubes, towards the egg.

For a baby to be made this way, the sperm cells must meet the egg on its way from the ovary to the uterus, in the fallopian tube.

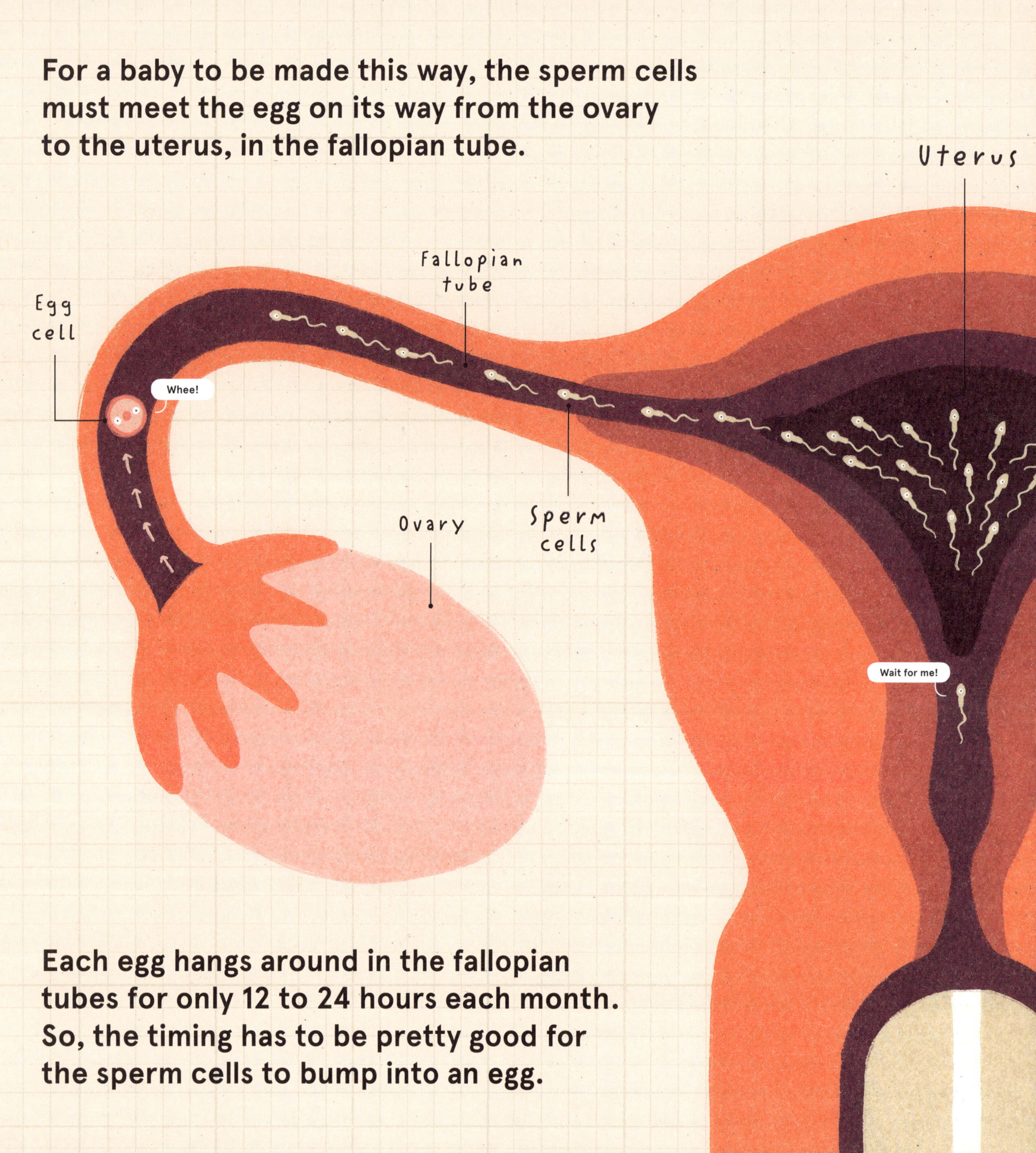

Each egg hangs around in the fallopian tubes for only 12 to 24 hours each month. So, the timing has to be pretty good for the sperm cells to bump into an egg.

Of the millions of sperm cells in the running, only one can win the race to enter the egg.

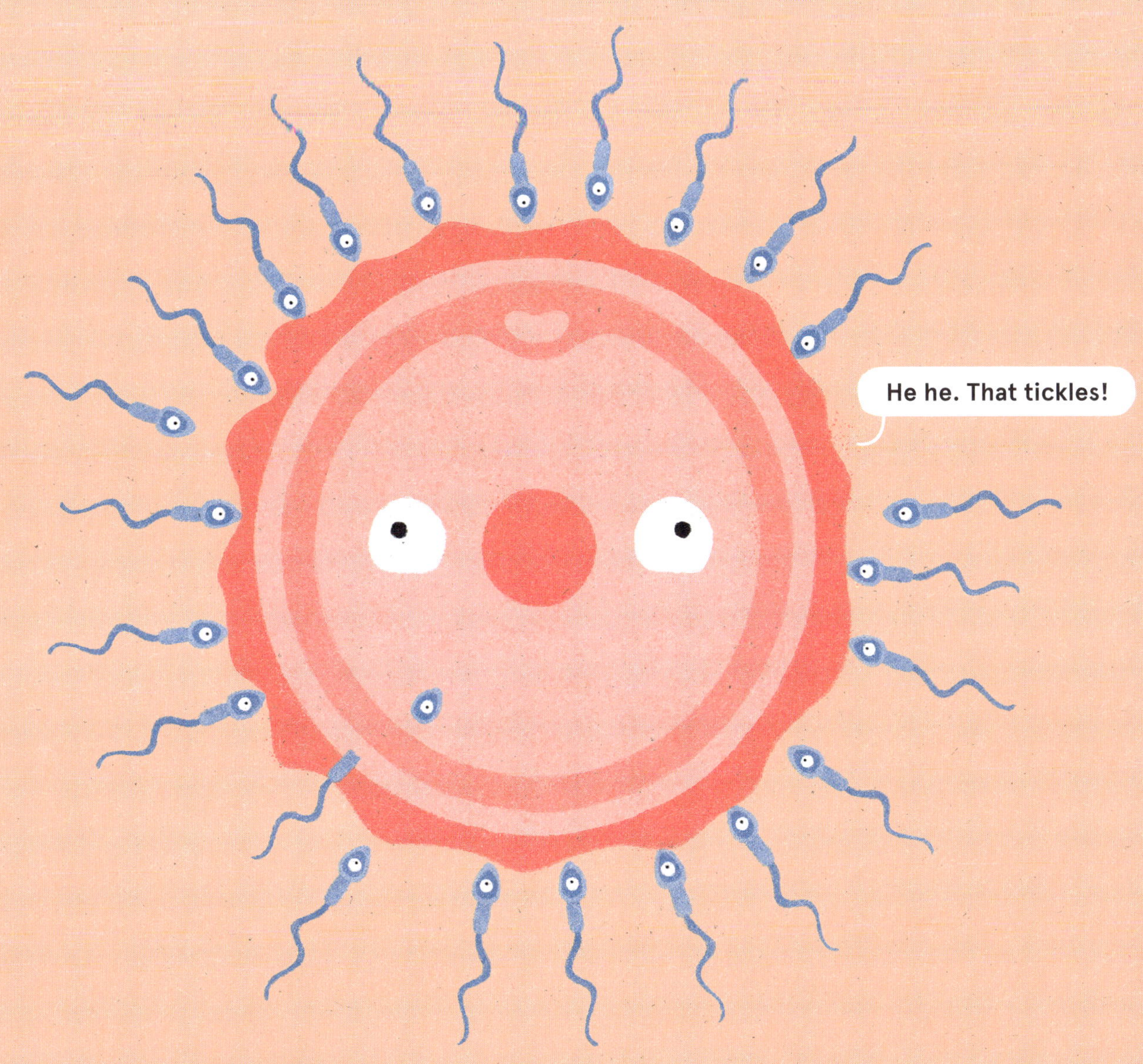

When the sperm cells finally meet the egg, the sperm must try to make their way through the outer layer of the egg. Once the first sperm makes it inside, its nucleus breaks free to search for the egg's nucleus.

And if the two nuclei successfully merge ...

Ta-da!

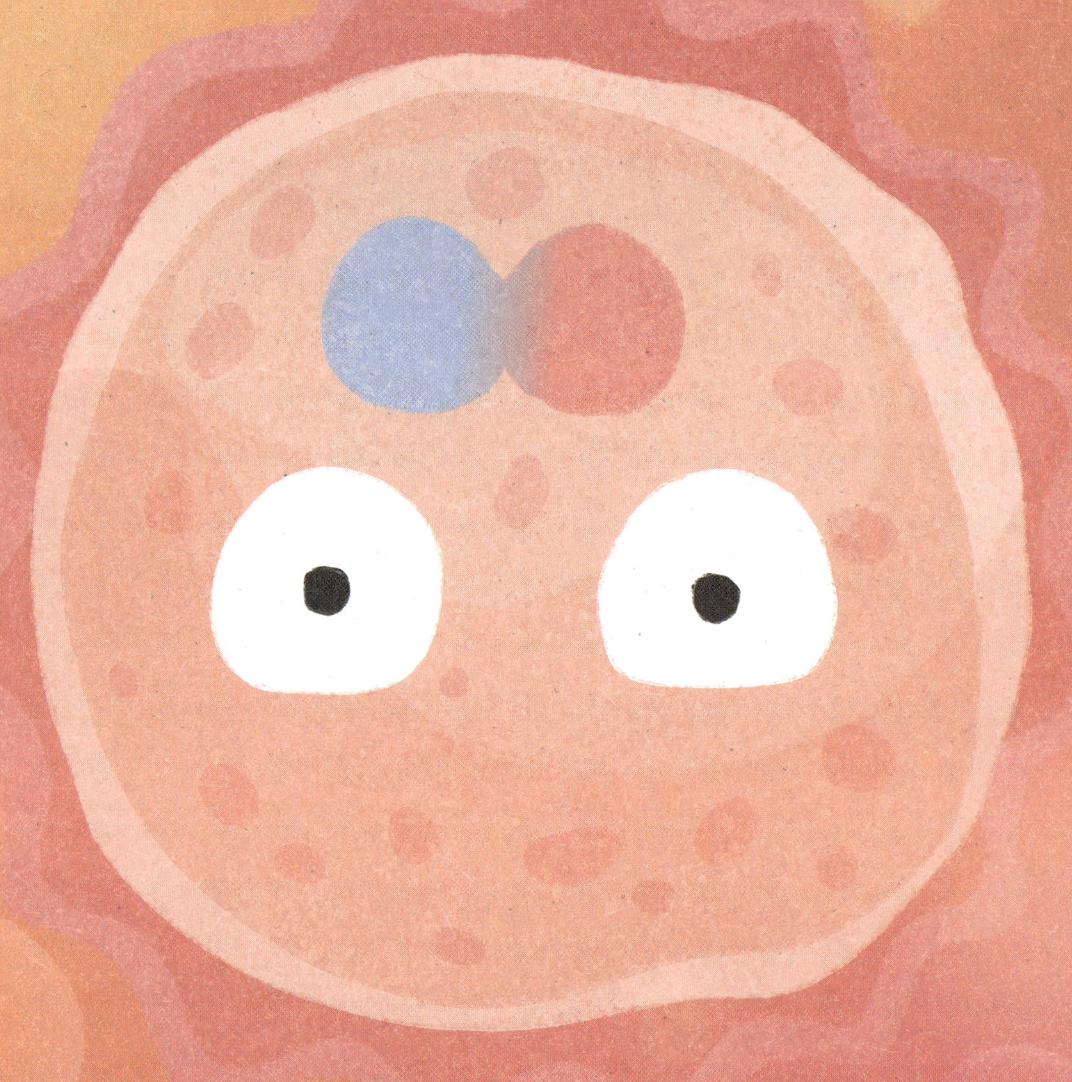

All of the stuff needed to make a baby is now held within that brilliant, beautiful ball. This is known as Fertilisation.

Once fertilised, the egg (who now goes by the rather spiffy name of 'Zygote') moves down the fallopian tube and into the uterus. From day one, the zygote begins to grow.

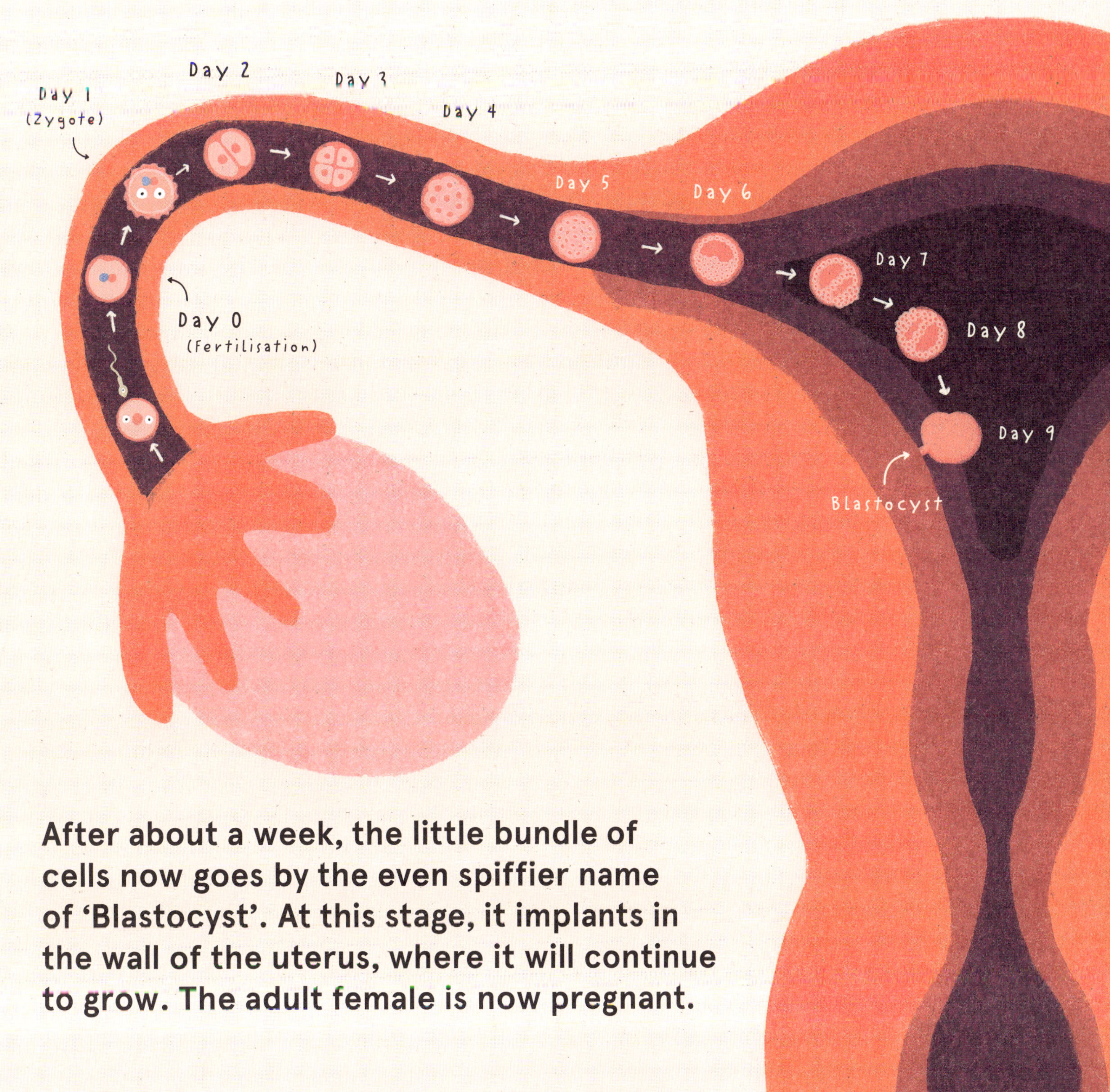

After about a week, the little bundle of cells now goes by the even spiffier name of 'Blastocyst'. At this stage, it implants in the wall of the uterus, where it will continue to grow. The adult female is now pregnant.

Sometimes adults very much want to have a baby, but they can't. There are heaps of reasons why many adults find it tough to make a baby. Sometimes the sperm aren't swimming, at other times there might be a problem with the eggs.

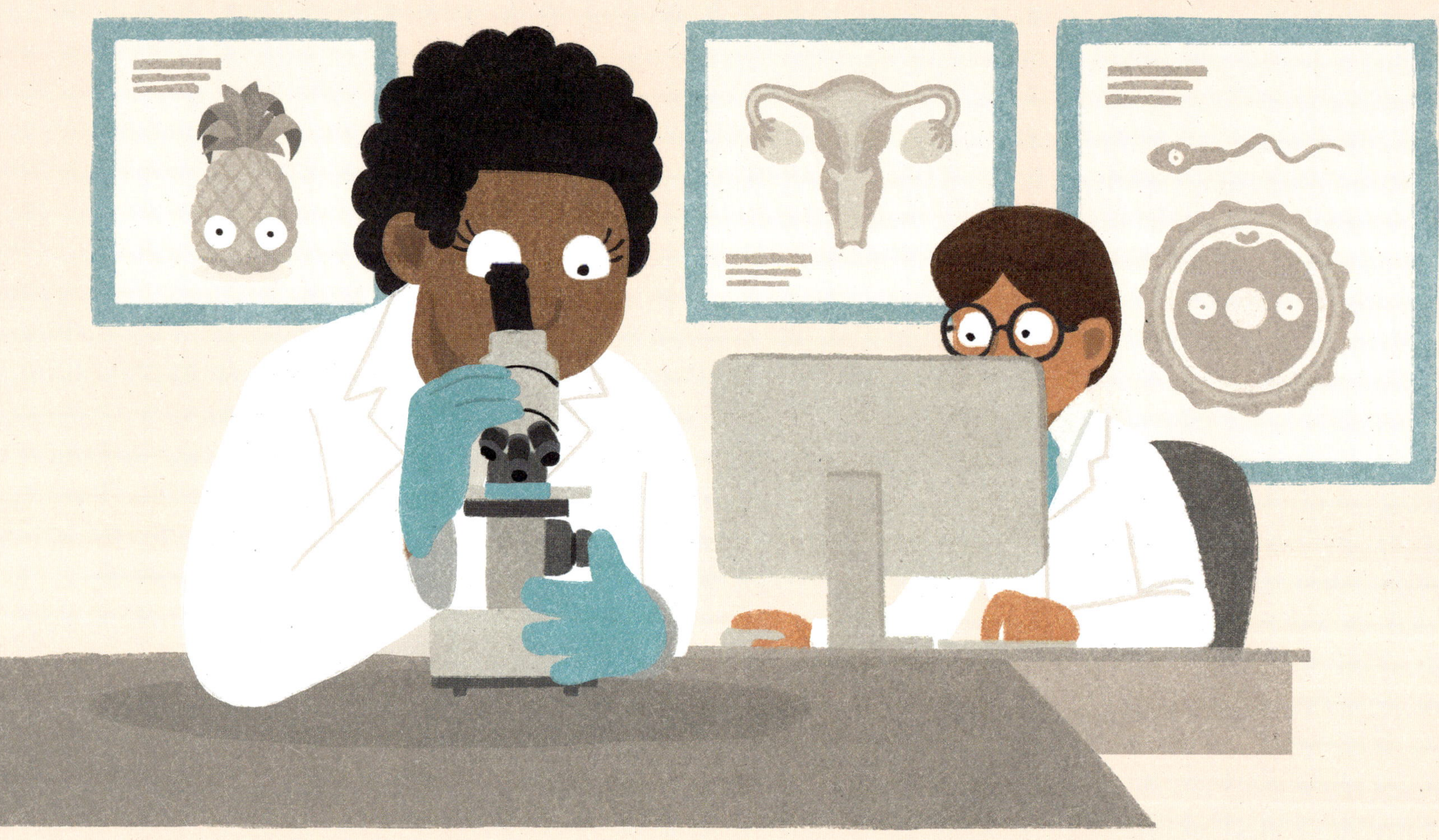

But we are lucky enough to live in a time and place where doctors know how to help people make babies.

One form of help is known as in vitro fertilisation (IVF). To begin this process, sperm and egg cells are collected from the biological father and mother.

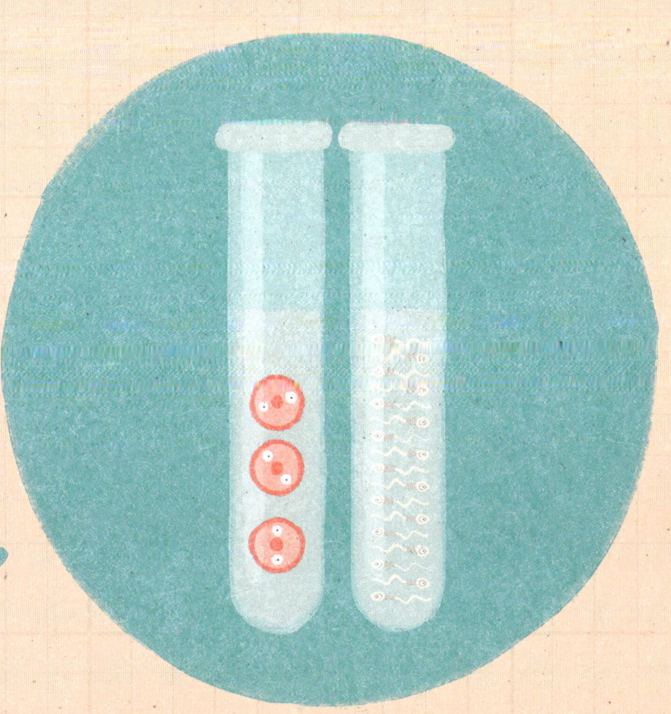

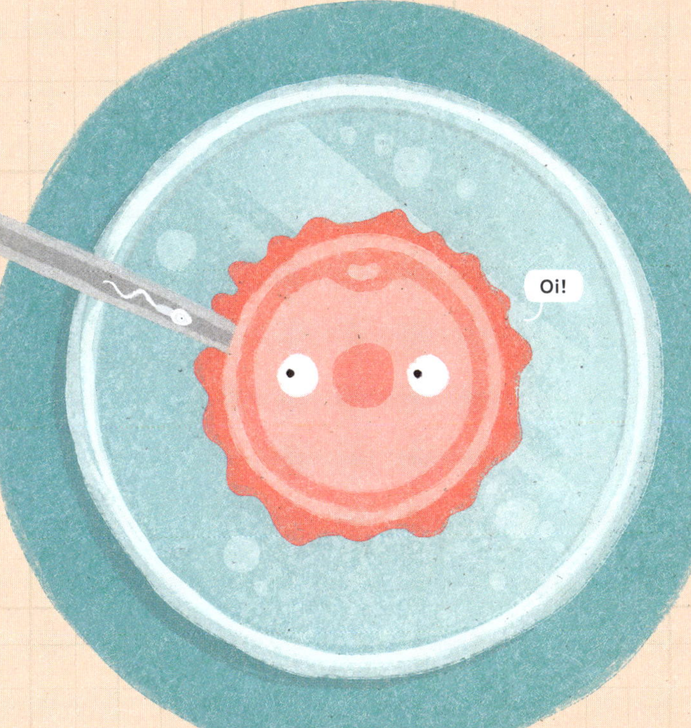

Fertility doctors introduce the sperm cells to the egg cells in a laboratory.

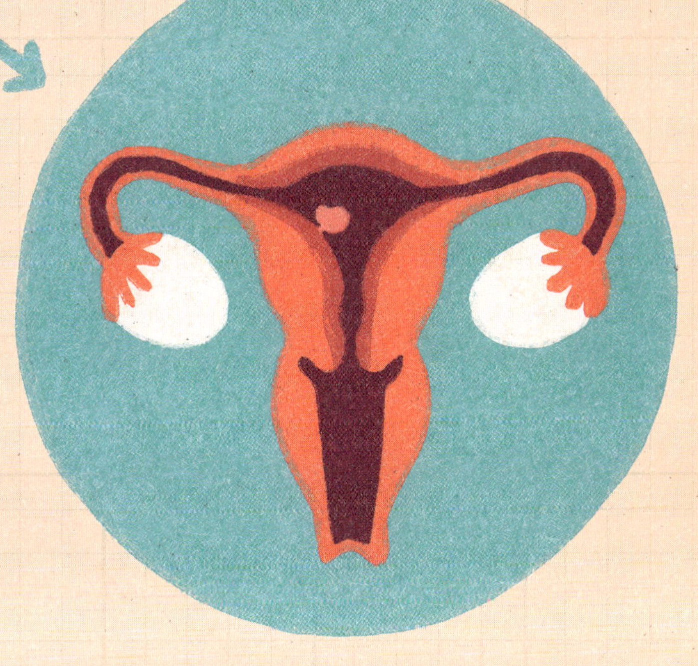

The fertilised egg is carefully placed into the uterus of the person who will carry the baby. All going well, the blastocyst will implant into the wall of the uterus, and away we go ...

Now, back to our little proto-person, who is comfortably hanging out on the wall of the uterus. After around 10 to 12 days, that little bundle of cells becomes an embryo.

Embr-yo!
4 weeks
(Poppy seed)
<1 mm
5 weeks
(Peppercorn)
~2 mm
6 weeks
(Pea)
~4 mm
7 weeks
(Blueberry)
~10 mm
8 weeks
(Raspberry)
~16 mm
9 weeks
(Olive)
~23 mm
10 weeks
(Prune)
~31 mm

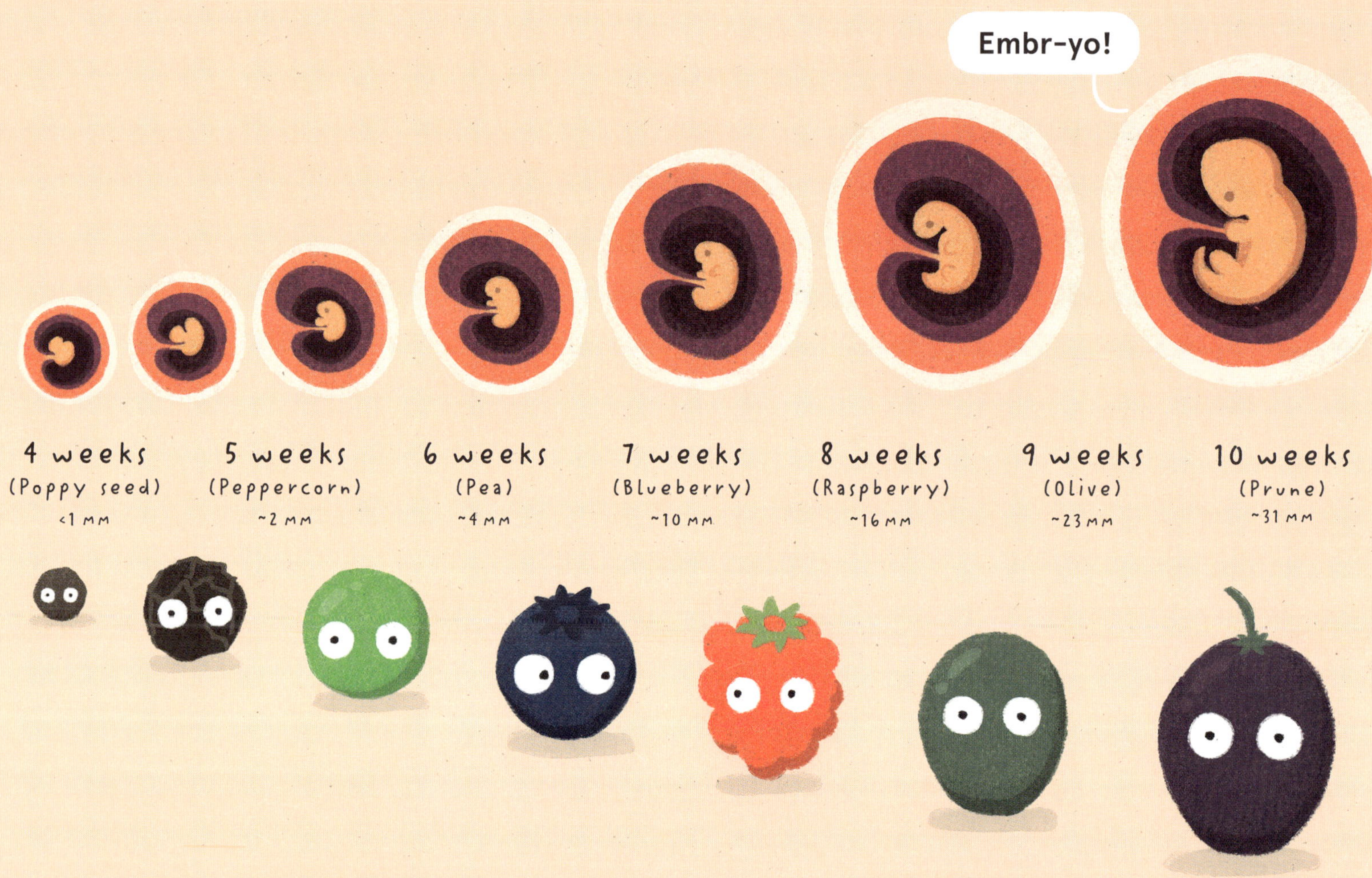

At around this point, doctors particularly enjoy comparing the growing embryo's size to various items from the supermarket (usually fruits and vegetables).

Occasionally, more than one baby can grow in the same uterus! A fertilised egg can split into two soon after fertilisation. When this happens, identical twins begin to grow in the uterus.

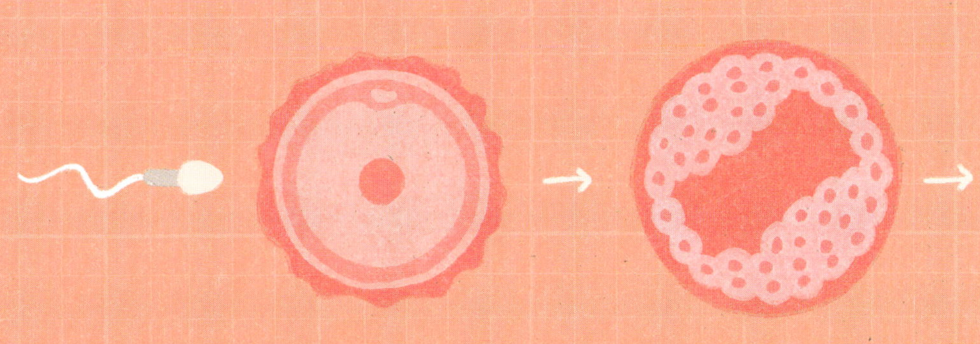

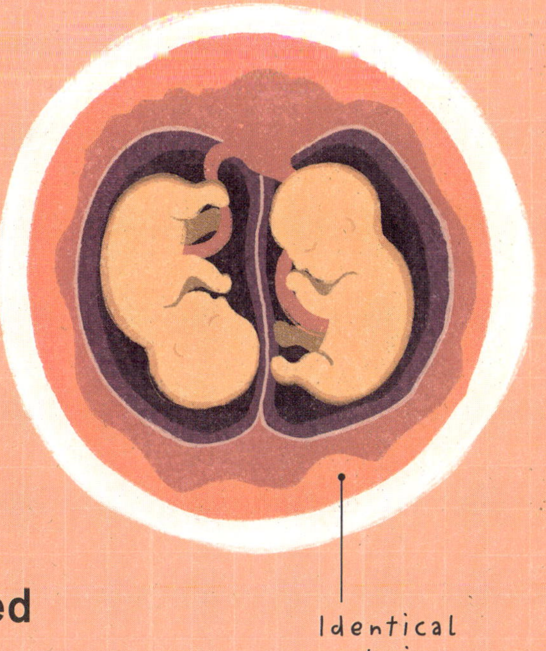

Every so often, two eggs are released from the ovaries. If both eggs are fertilised by sperm, non-identical twins can begin to grow in the uterus.

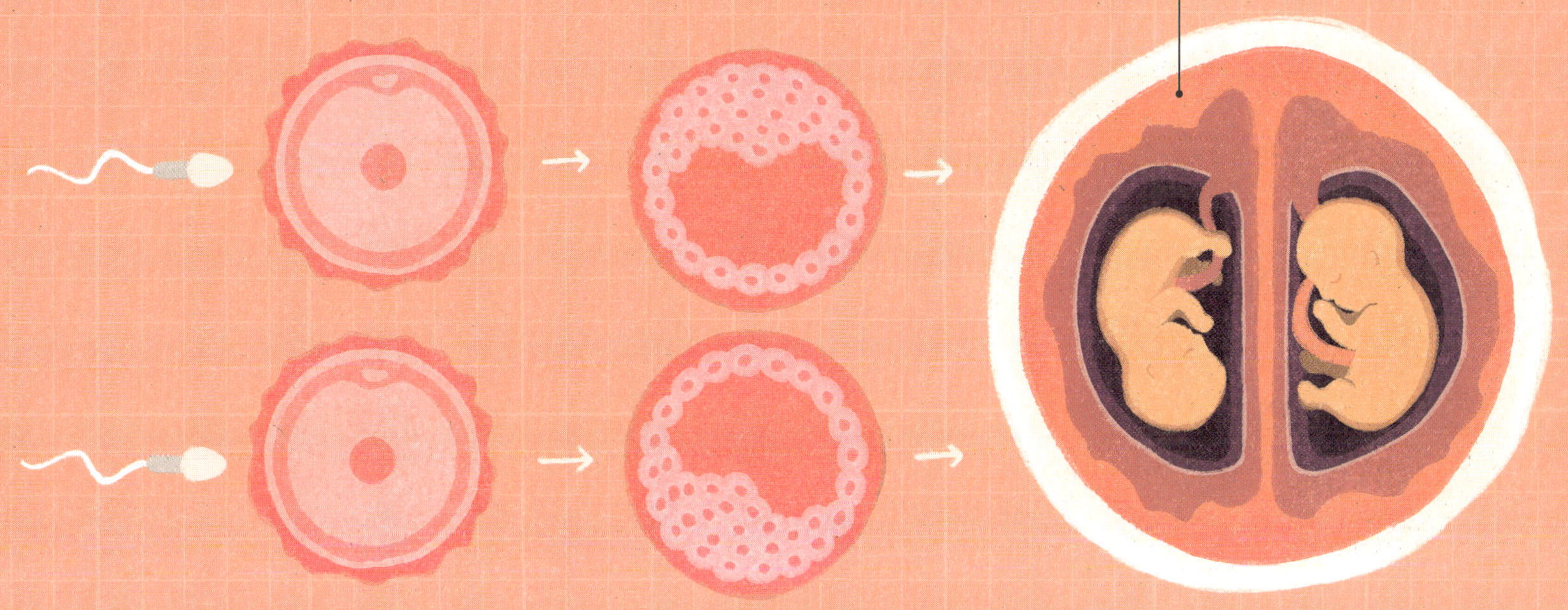

After a few months on the inside, the growing embryo is beginning to grow a little tired of being compared to groceries (and is now known as a foetus).

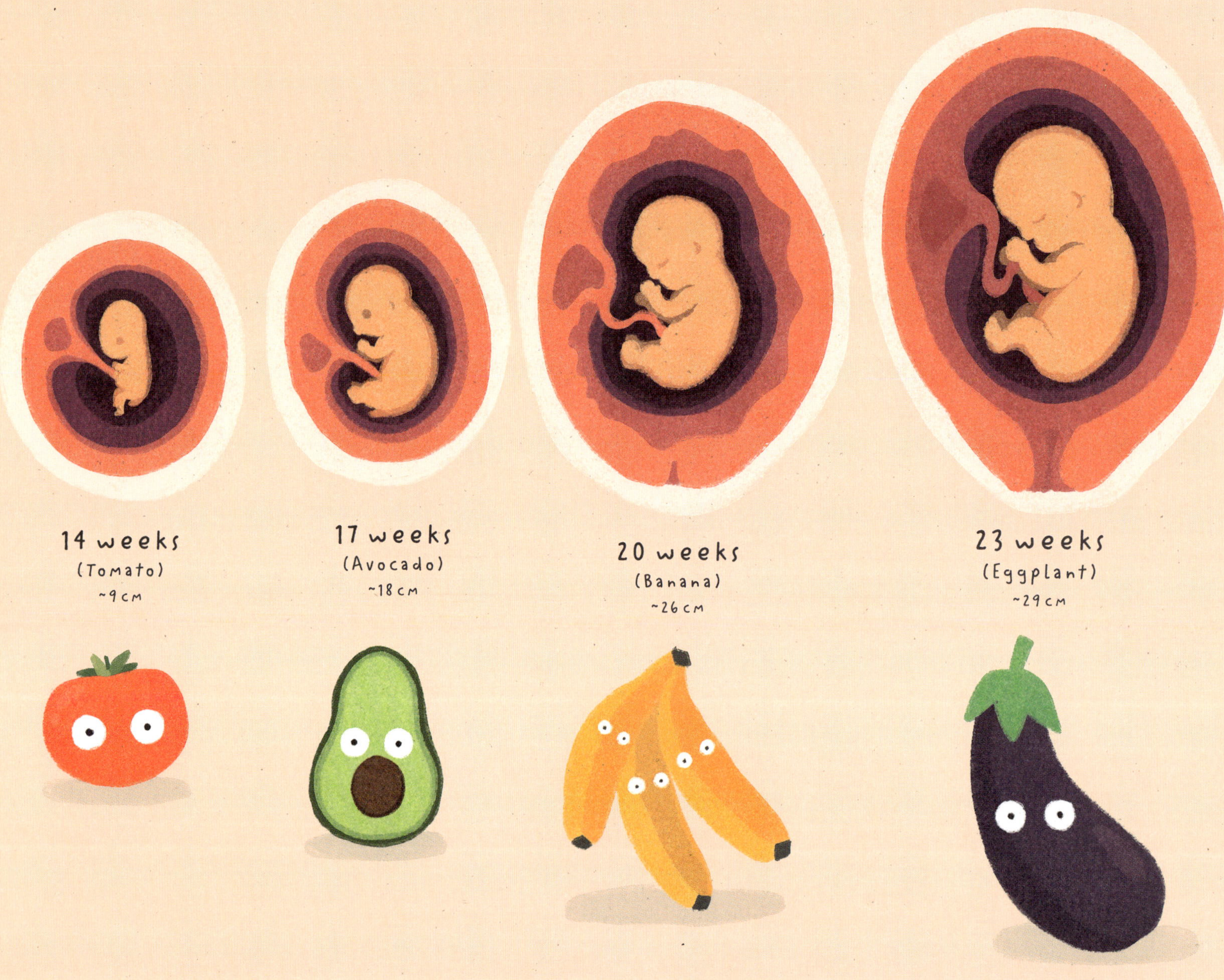

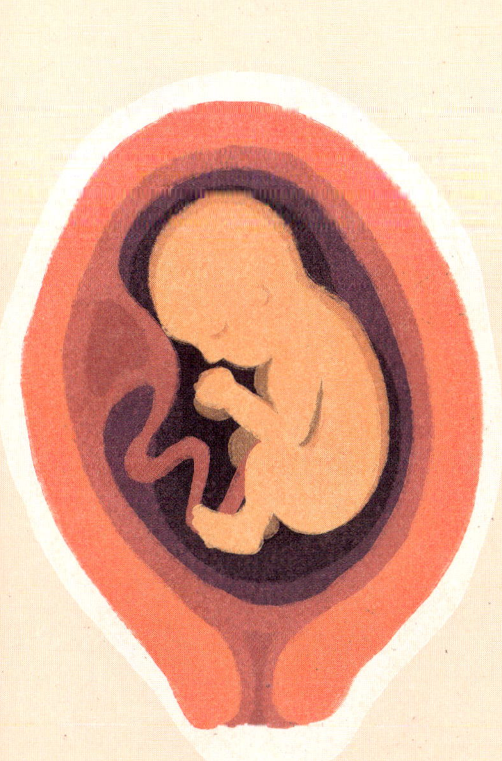

26 weeks
(Coconut)
~36 cm

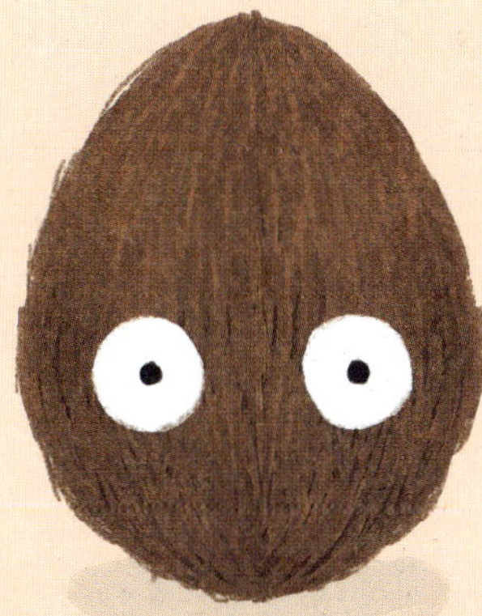

29 weeks
(Cabbage)
~39 cm

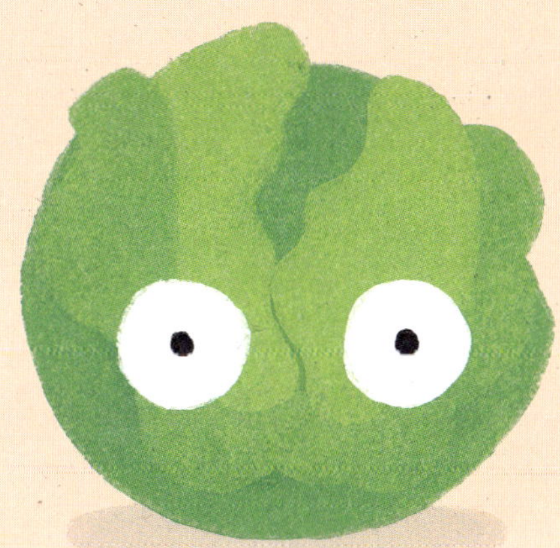

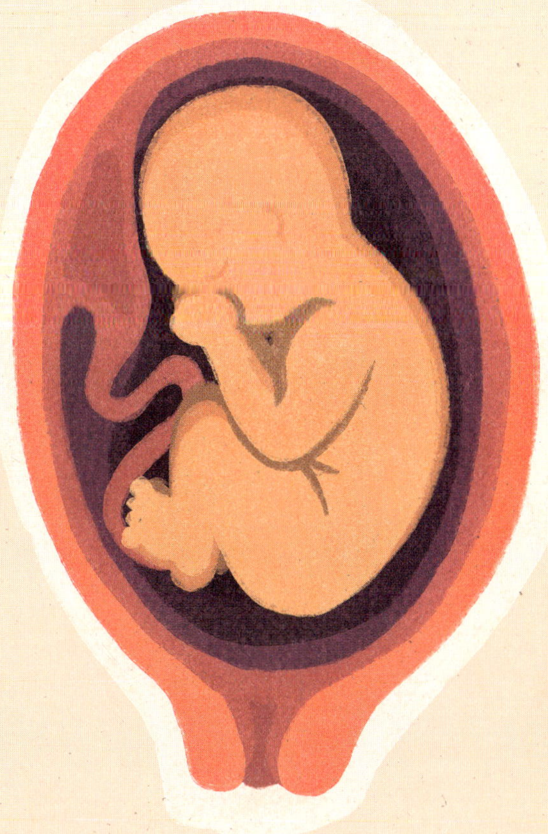

32 weeks
(Pineapple)
~42 cm

During the first three months of the pregnancy, the person carrying the baby develops a special organ within the uterus, called the placenta.

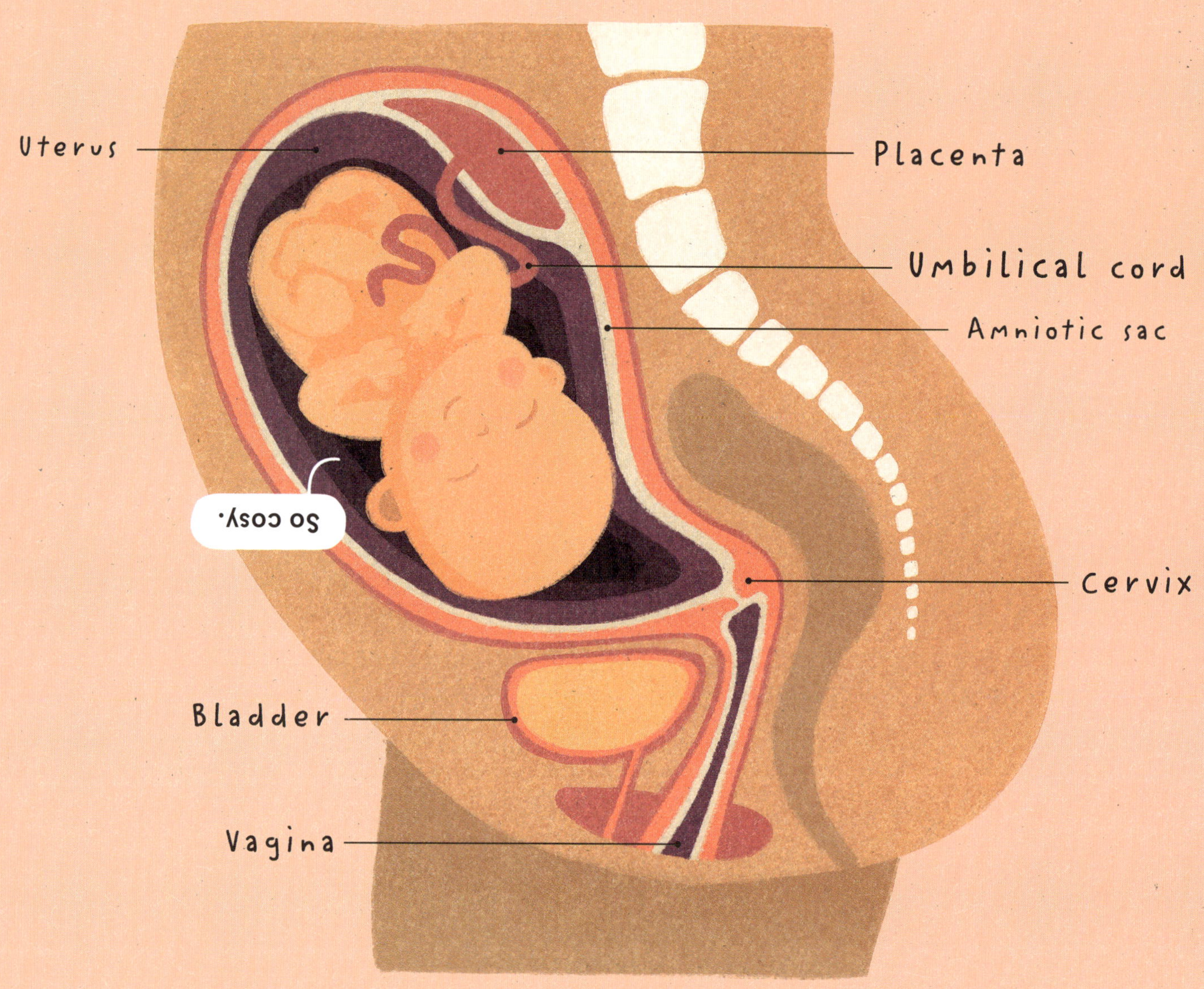

The placenta feeds the foetus through that ropey connection known as the umbilical cord.

A fluid-filled pouch called the amniotic sac helps protect the growing baby, and keep the temperature *just right*.

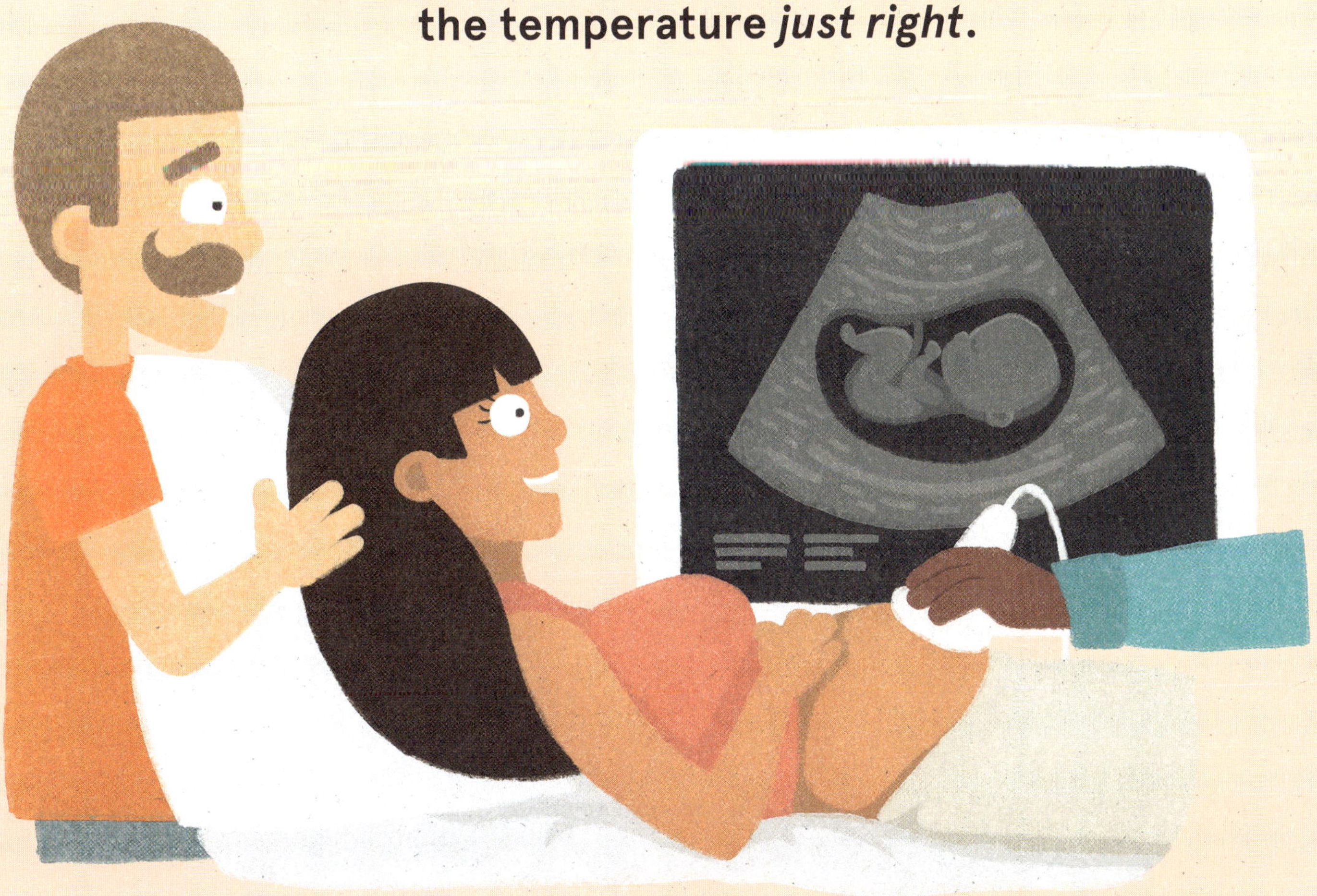

While they can pop out earlier, the baby is typically ready to be born after about 37 to 40 weeks on the inside. Or in the fancy-pants terminology of obstetrics … when the foetus is about the size of a watermelon.

40 weeks
(watermelon)
~51 cm

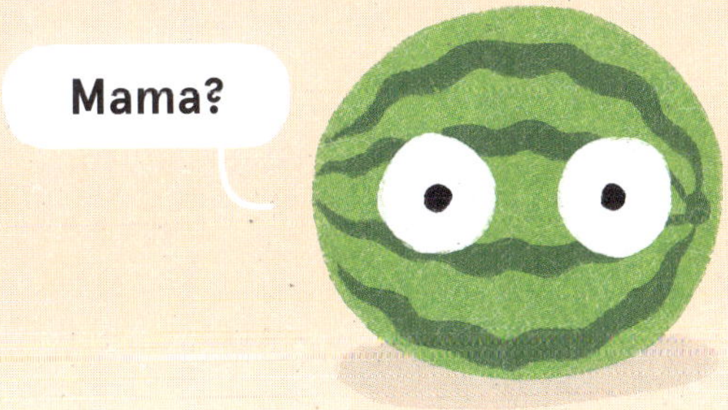

When the big day arrives, the female's body sends signals to the muscles around her uterus, which begin to tighten.

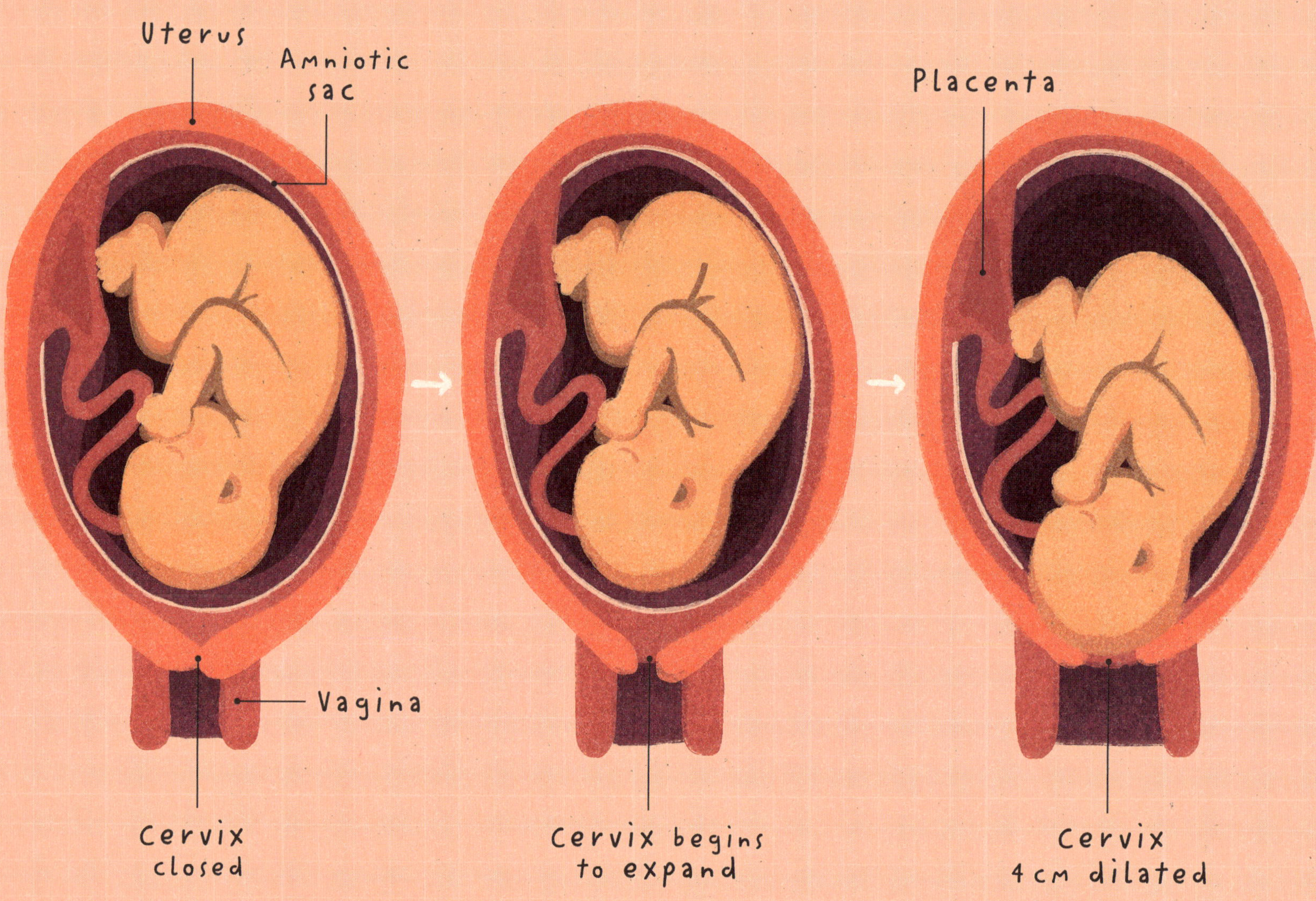

At the lower end, the cervix (the opening to her uterus) begins to expand.

These actions, known as contractions, begin to push the baby down from the uterus, through the vagina and out into the world.

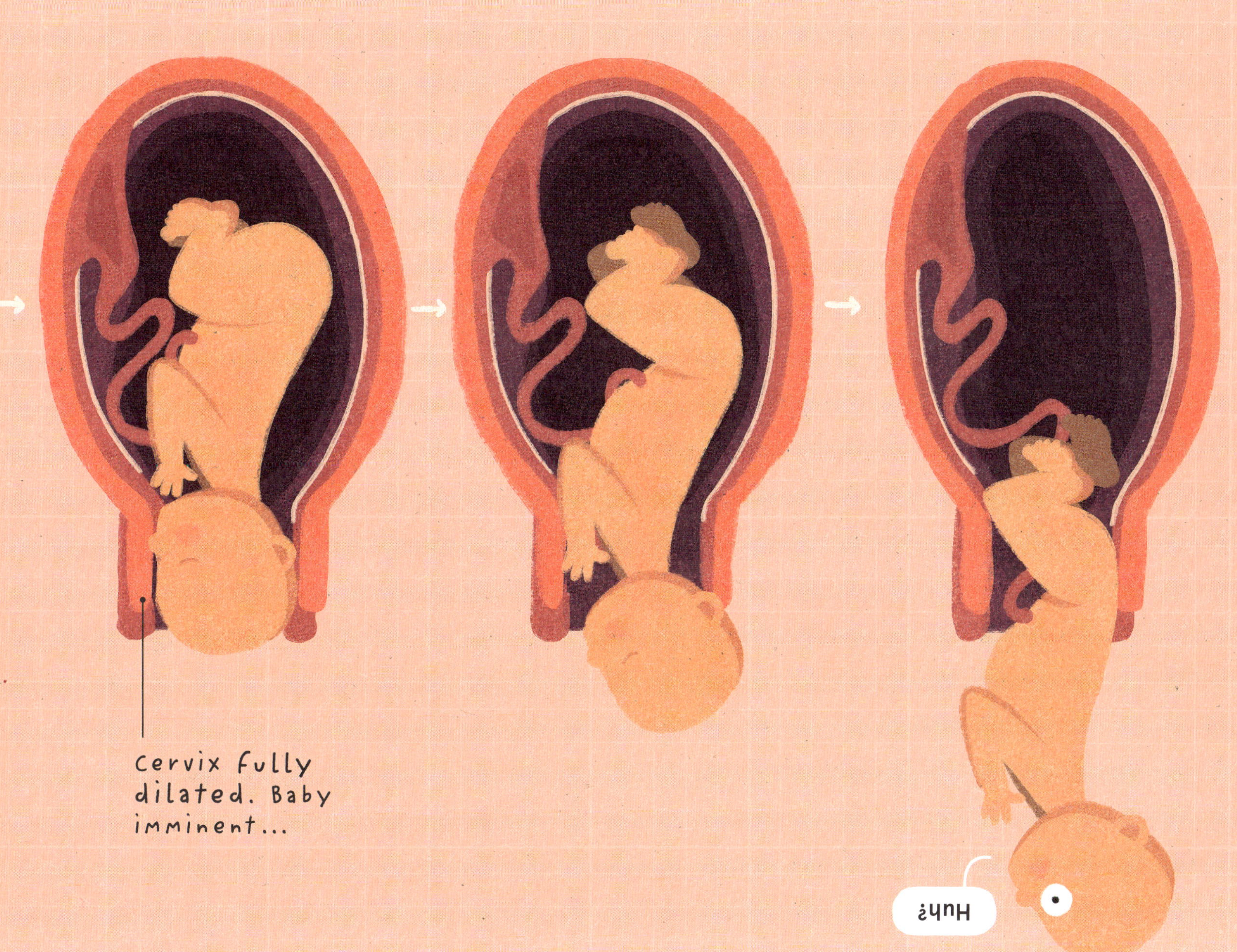

For a number of reasons, the pregnant person (or their doctors) might decide to bring the baby into the world in a slightly different way.

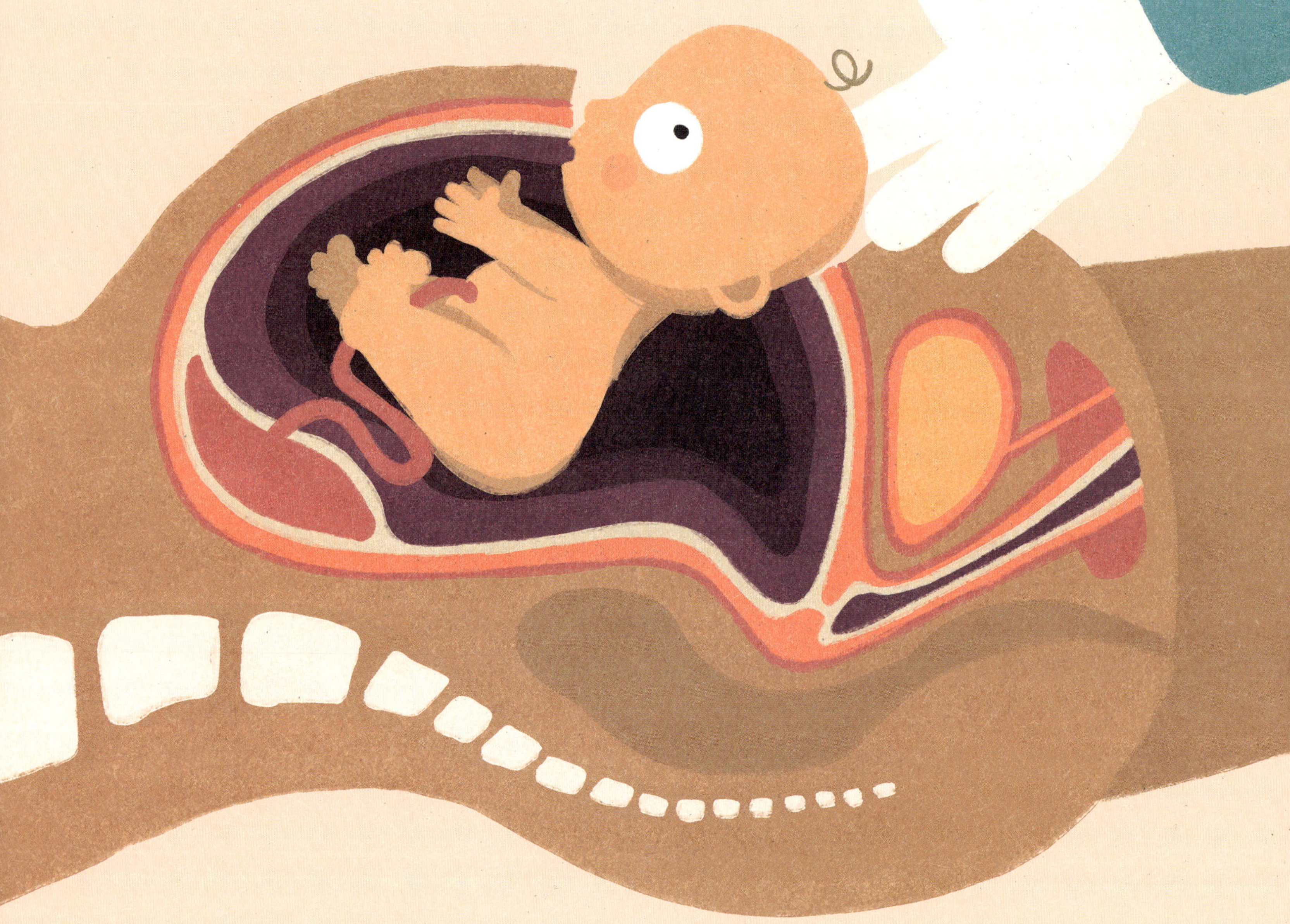

In a caesarean birth, doctors make a cut into the uterus. They remove the baby from the uterus through the cut, rather than through the vagina. The cut is then stitched back together and heals over time.

Either way, the baby leaves the uterus with the umbilical cord still attached to the placenta. Once the new baby emerges, they take their first breath, and the umbilical cord is cut.

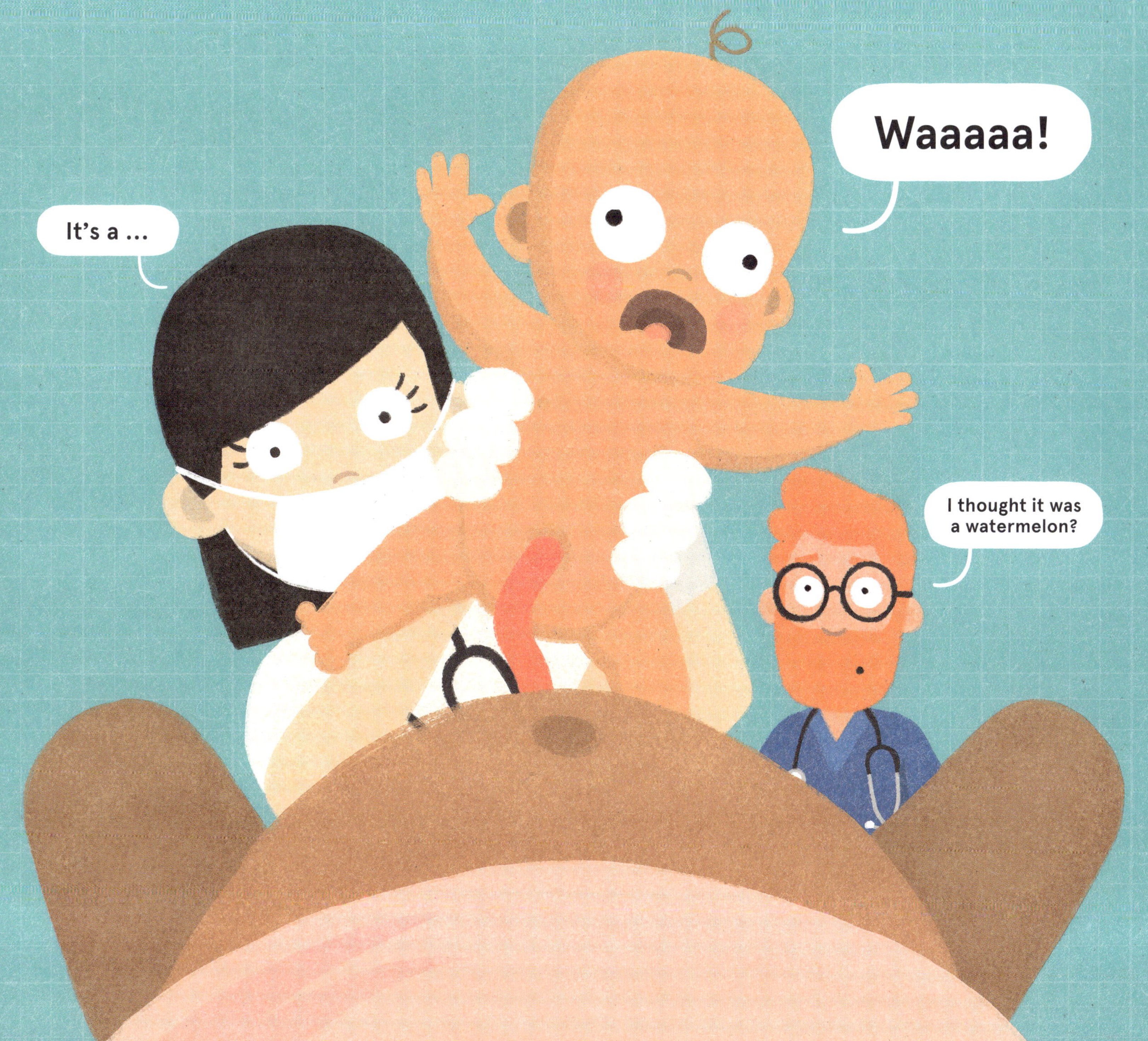

After all that, it's time to bond! Right about now, the baby might take their first few sips of milk, which is produced in the mother's breasts.

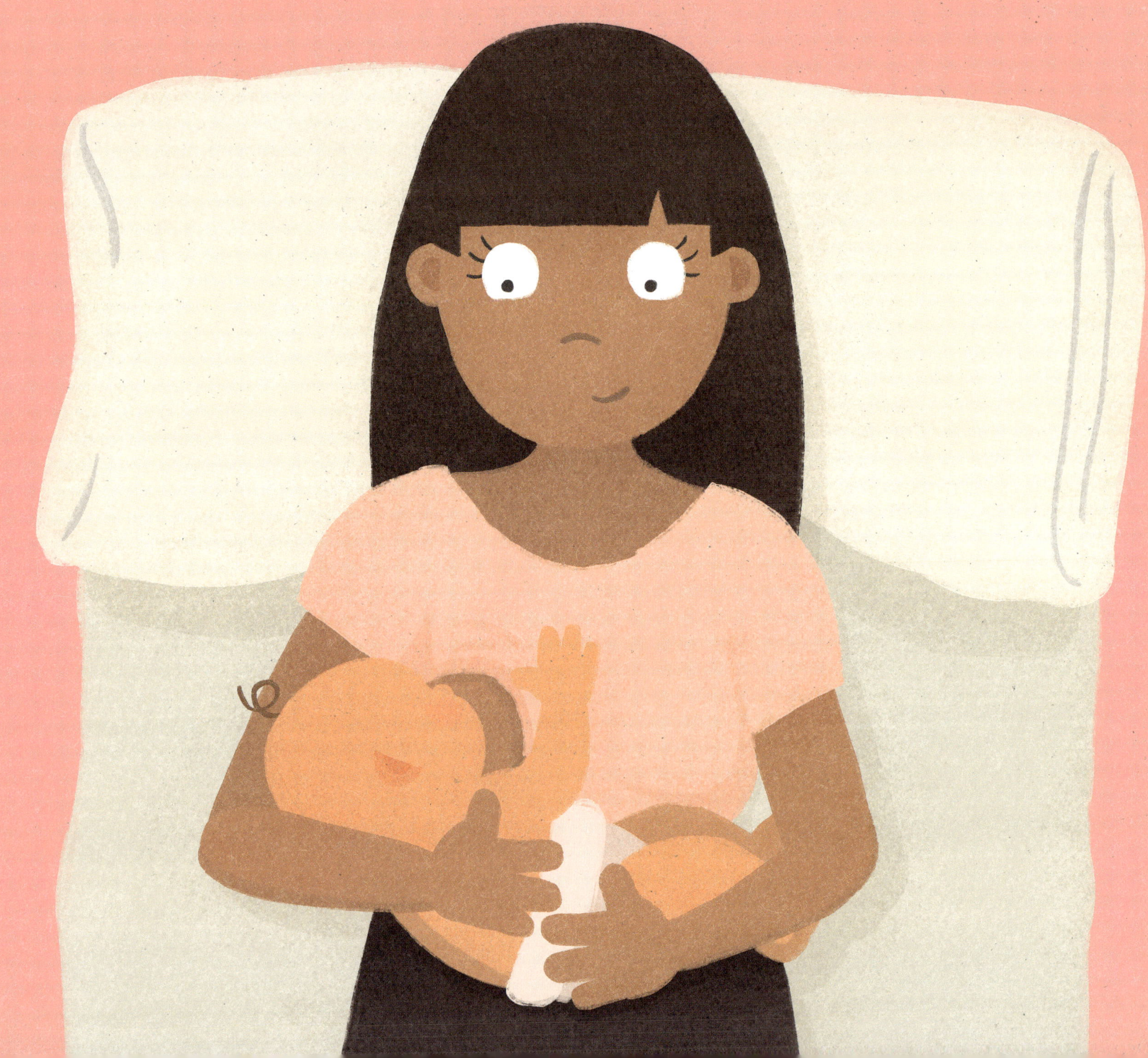

And that is how babies are made.

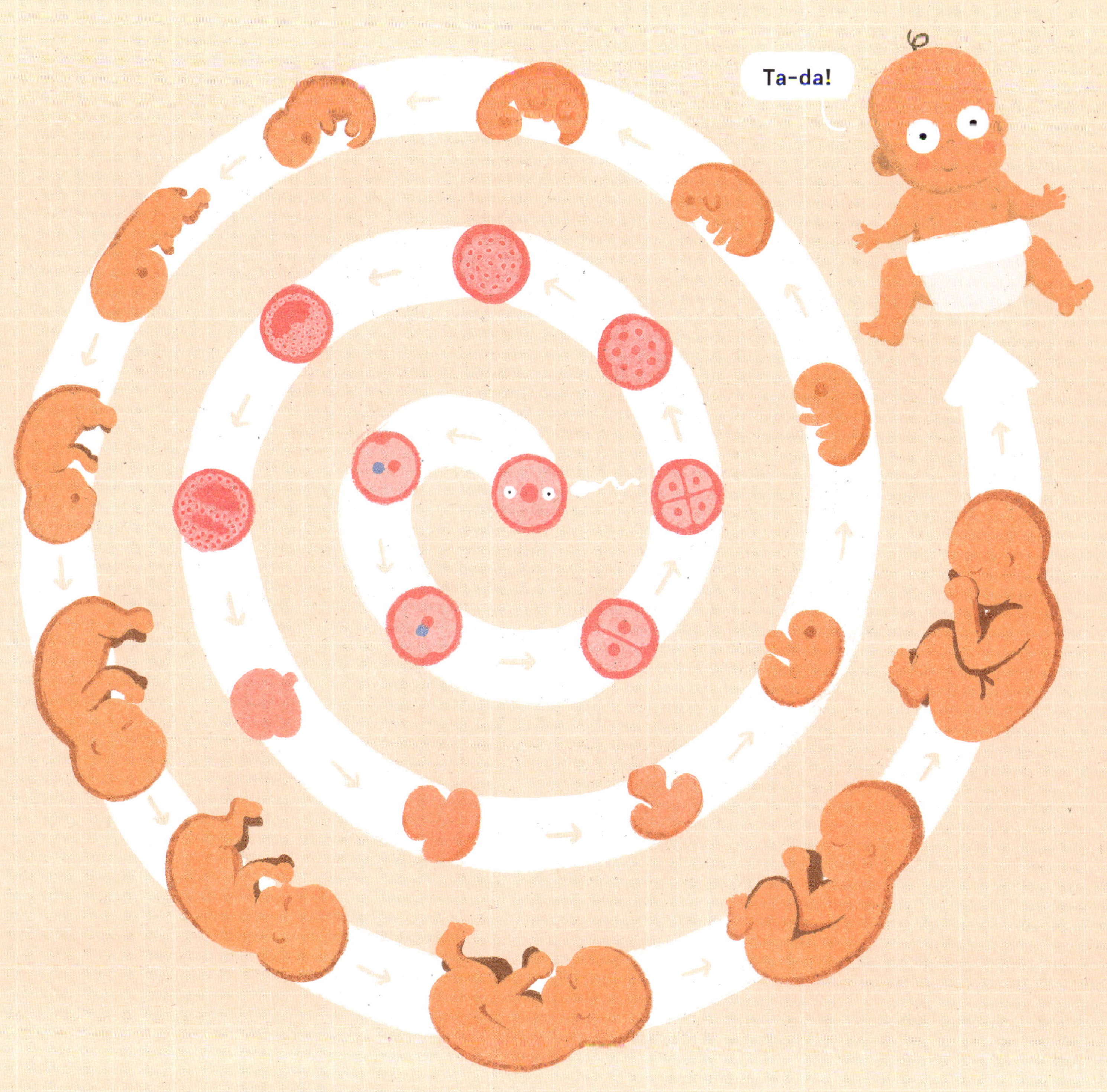

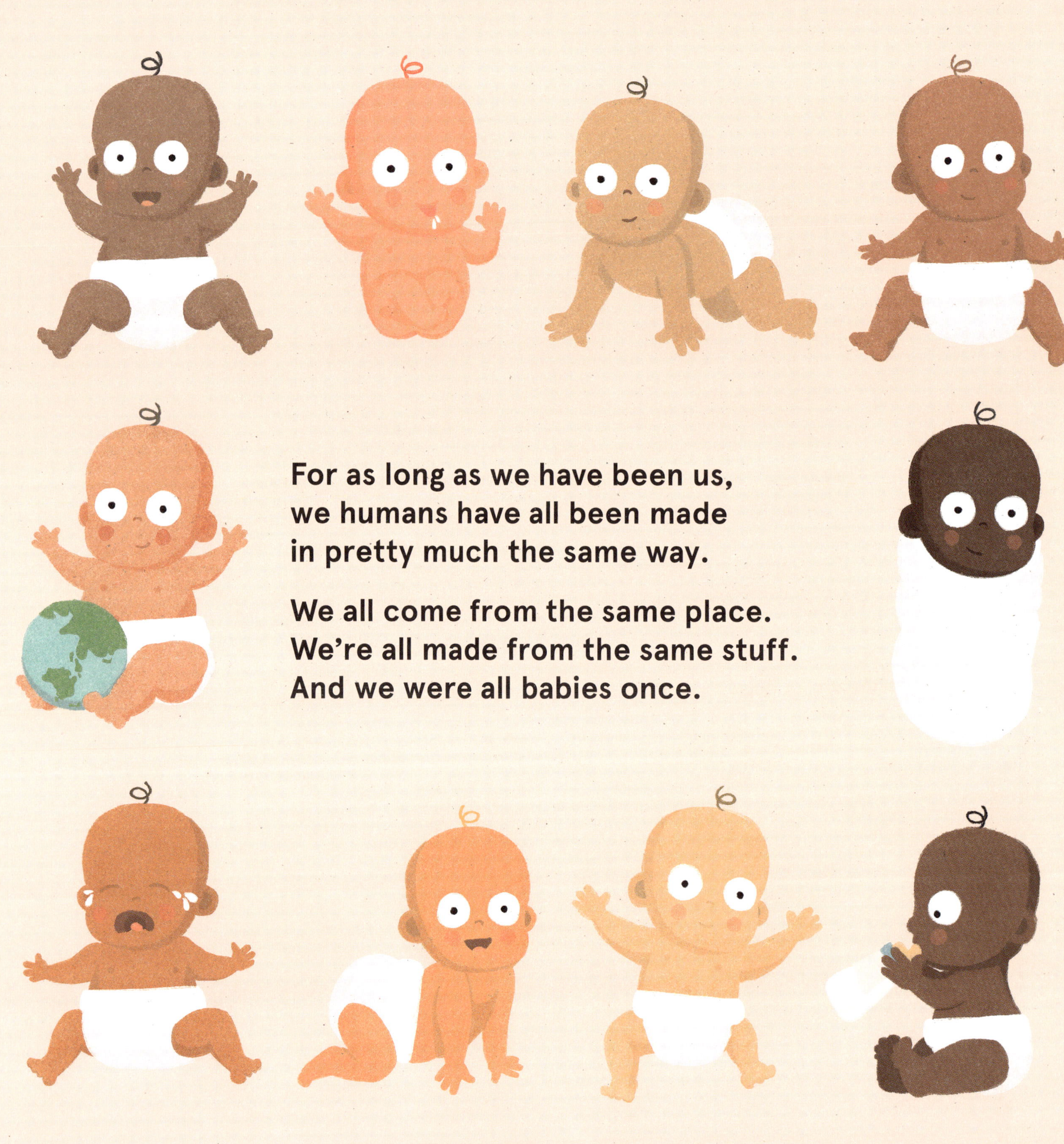

For as long as we have been us,
we humans have all been made
in pretty much the same way.

We all come from the same place.
We're all made from the same stuff.
And we were all babies once.

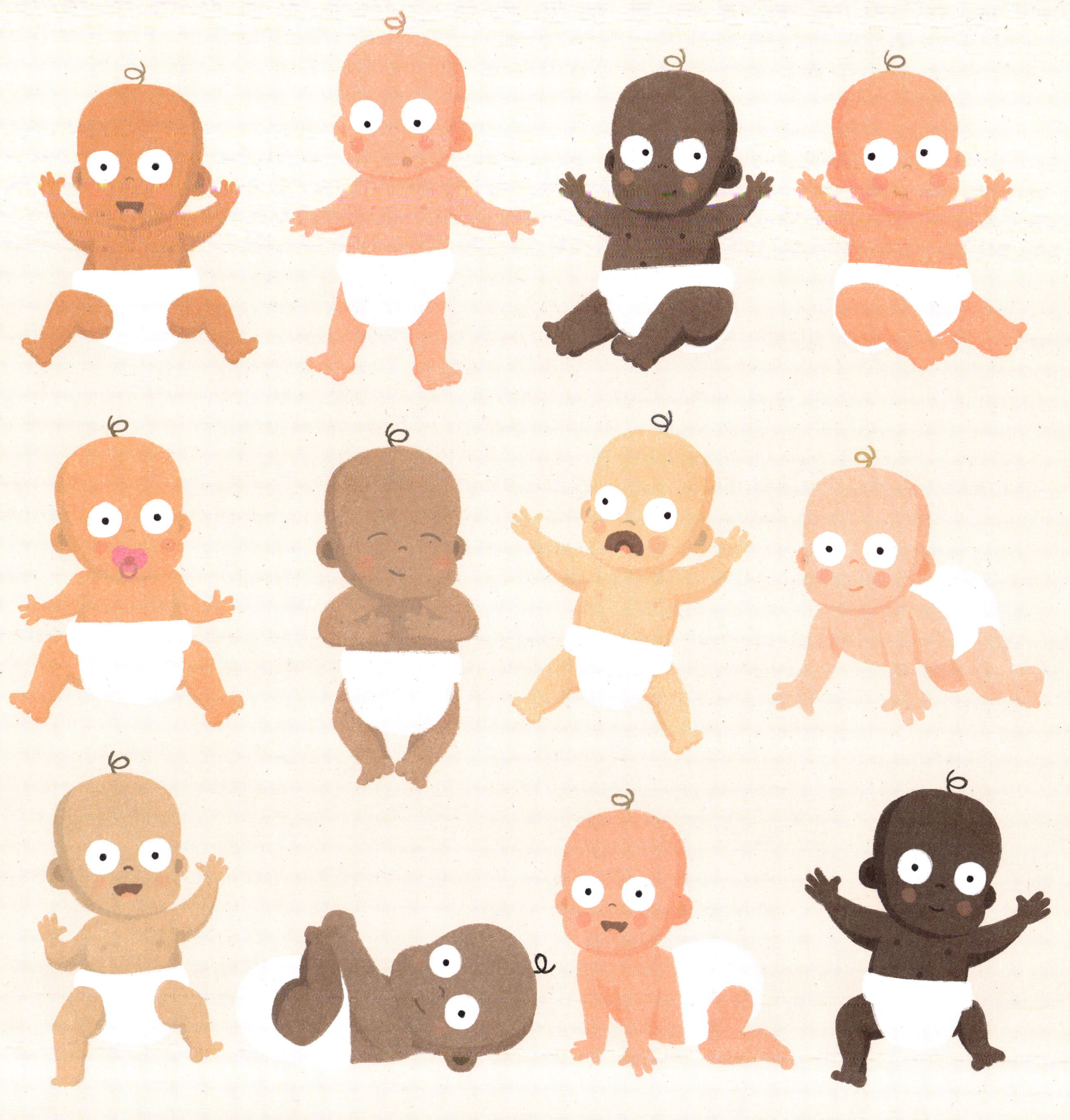

“The elegance of honesty needs no adornment.”

Mary Browne.

Scholastic Australia Pty Ltd
(ABN 11 000 614 577)
PO Box 579, Gosford NSW 2250.
www.scholastic.com.au

Part of the Scholastic Group
Sydney • Auckland • New York • Toronto • London • Mexico City •
New Delhi • Hong Kong • Buenos Aires • Puerto Rico

Published by Scholastic Australia in 2024.

Foreword by Dr Cindy Pan.

A catalogue record for this book is available from the National Library of Australia

ISBN: 978-1-76112-627-7 (hardback)

Printed in China by RR Donnelley. Scholastic Australia’s policy, in association with RR Donnelley, is to use papers that are renewable and made efficiently from wood grown in responsibly managed sources, so as to minimise its environmental footprint.

I acknowledge the traditional custodians of the land on which I live and work, and I pay respect to the Gubbi Gubbi nation. I pay respects to the Elders of the community and extend my recognition to their descendants. Philip Bunting

10 9 8 7 6 5 4 3 2 25 26 27 28 29 / 2

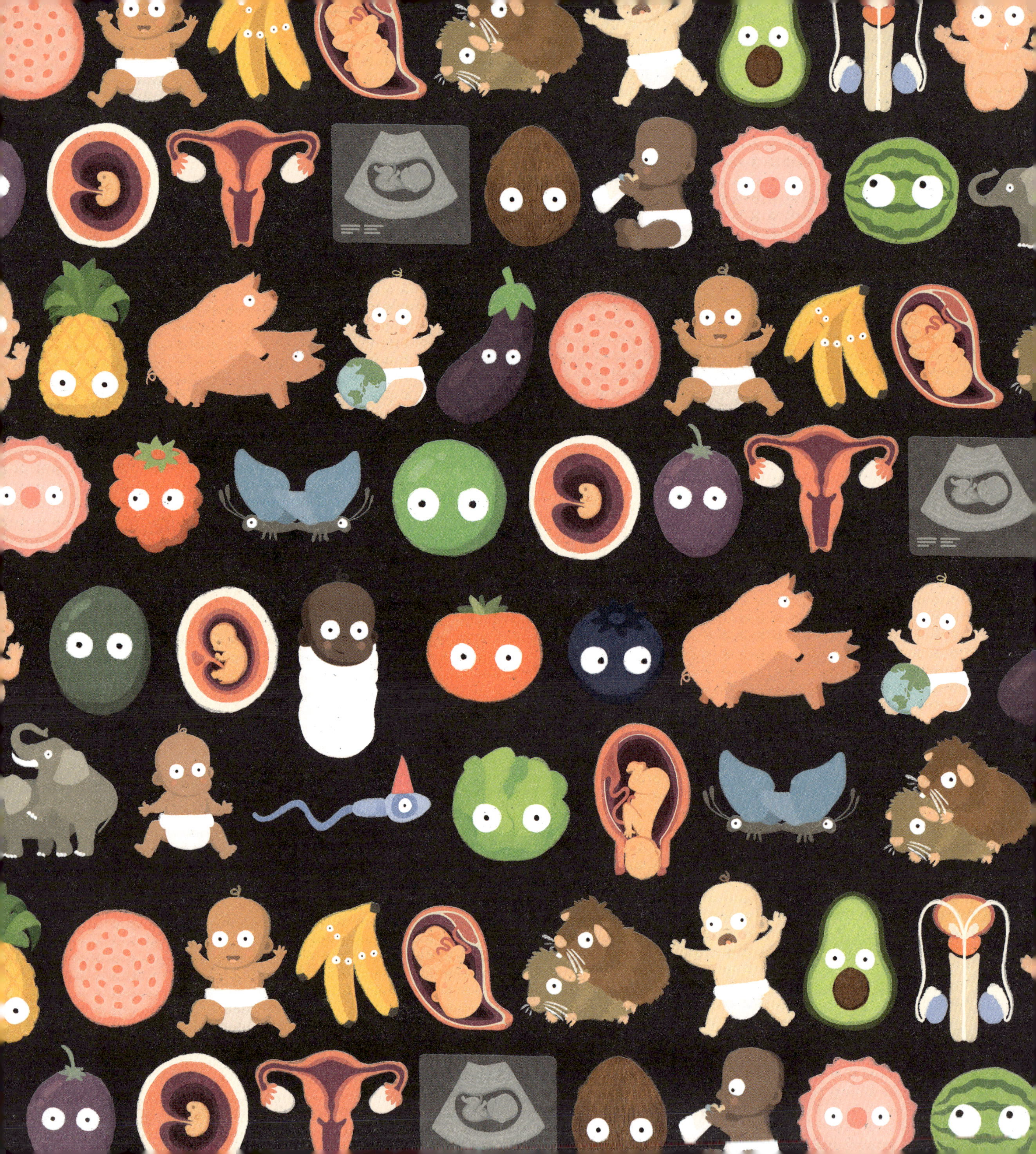